GRAINGER & ALLISON'S DIAGNOSTIC RADIOLOGY

SIXTH EDITION

The Spine

GRAINGER & ALLISON'S DIAGNOSTIC RADIOLOGY

The Spine

SIXTH EDITION

EDITED BY

Jonathan H. Gillard, BSc, MA, MD, FRCP, FRCR, MBA

H. Rolf Jäger, MD, FRCR

ELSEVIER

London   New York   Oxford   Philadelphia   St Louis   Sydney   Toronto

ELSEVIER

Executive Content Strategist: Michael Houston
Content Development Specialist: Louise Cook
Project Manager: Andrew Riley
Design: Christian Bilbow
Marketing Manager: Rachael Pignotti

Working together to grow libraries in developing countries

www.elsevier.com • www.bookaid.org

CONTENTS

PREFACE

The 6 chapters in this book have been selected from the contents of the Spine section in *Grainger & Allison's Diagnostic Radiology, Sixth Edition*. These chapters provide a succinct up-to-date overview of current imaging techniques and their clinical applications in daily practice and it is hoped that with this concise format the user will quickly grasp the fundamentals they need to know. Throughout these chapters, the relative merits of different imaging investigations are described, variations are discussed and recent imaging advances are detailed.

Grainger & Allison's Diagnostic Radiology has long been recognized as the standard general reference work in the field, and it is hoped that this book, utilizing the content from the latest sixth edition of this classic reference work, will provide radiology trainees and practitioners with ready access to the most current information, written by internationally recognized experts, on what is new and important in the radiological diagnosis of disorders of the spine.

LIST OF CONTRIBUTORS

Farah Alobeidi, MA, MB BChir, MRCS, FRCR
Neuroradiology Fellow, Lysholm Department of
  Neuroradiology, The National Hospital for
  Neurology and Neurosurgery, London, UK

Danielle Balériaux, MD
Professor Emeritus, Neuroradiology, Hôpital Erasme
  ULB, Brussels, Belgium

Arthur M. De Schepper, MD, PhD†
Former Radiologist, Department of Radiology,
  University Hospital Antwerp, Edegem, Belgium

Jonathan H. Gillard, BSc, MA, MD, FRCP, FRCR, MBA
Professor of Neuroradiology, University of Cambridge,
  Addenbrooke's Hospital, Cambridge, UK

H. Rolf Jäger, MD, FRCR
Reader in Neuroradiology, Department of Brain Repair
  and Rehabilitation, UCL Institute of Neurology,
  UCL Faculty of Brain Sciences; Consultant
  Neuroradiologist, Lysholm Department of
  Neuroradiology, National Hospital for Neurology
  and Neurosurgery, and Department of Imaging,
  University College London Hospitals, London, UK

Tomasz Matys, PhD, FRCR
Specialist Registrar in Clinical Radiology;
  Neuroradiology Fellow, Addenbrooke's Hospital,
  Cambridge University Hospitals NHS Foundation
  Trust, Cambridge, UK

Paul M. Parizel, MD, PhD
Professor and Chair, Department of Radiology,
  Antwerp University Hospital, University of Antwerp,
  Edegem, Belgium

James J. Rankine, MB ChB, MRCP, MRaD, FRCR, MD
Consultant Radiologist and Honorary Clinical Associate
  Professor, Department of Radiology, Leeds General
  Infirmary, Leeds, West Yorkshire, UK

Nasim Sheikh-Bahaei, MD, MRCP, FRCR
Clinical Lecturer, University Department of Radiology,
  Cambridge University Hospitals NHS Foundation
  Trust, Cambridge, UK

Majda M. Thurnher, MD
Associate Professor of Radiology, Medical University
  Vienna, Department of Biomedical Imaging and
  Image-Guided Therapy, Vienna, Austria

Luc van den Hauwe, MD
Consultant Radiologist, Department of Radiology,
  University Hospital Antwerp, Edegem; Department
  of Radiology, AZ KLINA, Brasschaat, Belgium

Johan W. Van Goethem, MD, PhD
Vice Departmental Head, Department of Radiology
  and Neuroradiology, Antwerp University Hospital,
  Edegem, Belgium

Thomas Van Thielen, MD
Resident, Department of Radiology, University
  Hospital Antwerp, Edegem, Belgium

CHAPTER 1

IMAGING TECHNIQUES AND ANATOMY

Thomas Van Thielen • Luc van den Hauwe • Johan W. Van Goethem • Paul M. Parizel

CHAPTER OUTLINE

ANATOMY
Osseous Elements
Joints
Ligaments
Neural Structures—Spinal Cord,
    Spinal Nerves, Dura Mater
Vascular Structures
Craniocervical Junction

IMAGING TECHNIQUES
Plain Radiography
Myelography
Spinal Angiography
Computed Tomography
Magnetic Resonance Imaging

ANATOMY

Anatomically the spine is organised segmentally, consisting of 7 cervical, 12 thoracic, 5 lumbar, 5 (fused) sacral and 3–5 coccygeal vertebra. Each level, except C1, consists out of the following elements: a vertebral body (corpus vertebrae) anteriorly and a vertebral or neural arch (arcus posterior) posteriorly. Together these two structures enclose the spinal canal.

Functionally the spine can be divided in three so-called columns.[1] The anterior column includes the anterior longitudinal ligament, the anterior annulus fibrosus and the anterior two-thirds of the vertebral body. The middle column comprises the posterior third of the vertebral body, the posterior annulus fibrosus and the posterior longitudinal ligament. The posterior column includes the posterior elements with the pedicles, facet joints, laminae and spinous processes as well as the posterior ligaments.

OSSEOUS ELEMENTS

Vertebral Body

The vertebral bodies have a thin rim of cortical bone and a central framework of mostly vertically orientated trabeculae. This osseous portion contains stores of phosphate and calcium and has a structural support function. Sclerotic bands can be seen in the vertebral body at the site of fusion between two vertebral components. This is typically seen at the neurocentral junction and in the dens axis. In the dens axis there may be remnants of the subdental synchondrosis. These bony structures are optimally evaluated with computed tomography (CT) imaging and to a lesser extent with magnetic resonance

imaging (MRI). On CT imaging vascular channels are often visible and in a post-traumatic setting can be mistaken for small fractures.

The centre of the vertebral body is composed of red bone marrow, which is haematopoietically active. Red and yellow bone marrow are not entirely homogeneous and each contain elements of the other. The vertebral marrow is dynamic, changing with age, immune state, oxygenation, coagulation and structural needs.[2] The normal adult distribution of bone marrow is reached by the age of 25. With ageing, the bone marrow assumes a more variable appearance with a reduction in the red cell mass and trabecular bone and increase of the fatty content. These changes appear relatively late in comparison to the changes in the bone marrow in the peripheral skeleton. The distribution of the red bone marrow in a vertebral body is predominantly seen at the metaphyseal equivalents near the endplates and the anterior part of the vertebra.[3] Evaluation of the bone marrow is best done with MRI. In the normal spinal marrow the distribution patterns of fatty and red marrow were categorised into four patterns by Ricci and colleagues[4] (Fig. 1-1). Pattern 1 describes a uniform low signal on T_1–weighted images with high linear signal around the basivertebral vein; this type is most commonly seen in younger patients aged 30 or less. Type 2 is a band-like high T_1 signal limited to the periphery of the vertebral body. Type 3 is characterised by multiple small indistinct (difficult to visualise) high signal intensity foci on T_1-weighted images throughout the vertebral body. These two patterns (types 2 and 3) are seen with increasing age and typically in persons of 40 years and older. Type 4 is a more severe form of type 3 with multiple larger high signal intensity foci (5–15 mm) on T_1 images throughout the vertebral body.

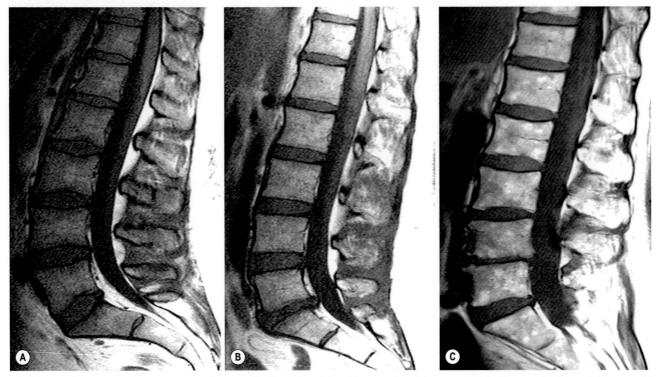

FIGURE 1-1 ■ **Age-related bone marrow changes.** Sagittal T_1-weighted images in a 23 year old (A), 44 year old (B) and 73 year old (C). Normal patterns of bone marrow distribution as described by Ricci and colleagues.[4] (A) Type 1 bone marrow pattern with uniform low signal intensity and a high linear signal around the basivertebral vein. (B) A type 2 pattern with band-like hyperintense signal intensity limited to the periphery and (C) a type 4 marrow pattern in a 73 year old with large hyperintense foci.

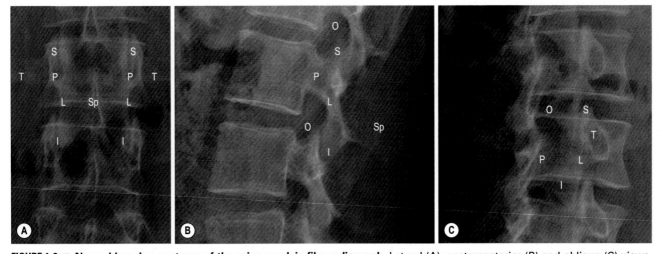

FIGURE 1-2 ■ **Normal imaging anatomy of the spine on plain film radiograph.** Lateral (A), posteroanterior (B) and oblique (C) views. P = pedicle, L = lamina, I = inferior articular process, S = superior articular process, Sp = spinous process, T = transverse process, O = intervertebral foramen.

Neural Arch

The neural arch, also known as posterior arch, forms the bony lateral and posterior border of the spinal canal (Figs. 1-2–1-4). It can be divided into different segments. Between the transverse and spinous process the neural arch is called the lamina. The pedicle is the part situated between the transverse process and the vertebral body. The pedicle of each vertebra is notched at its inferior and superior edge. Together these notches form an opening called the intervertebral foramen. Through this foramen the spinal nerves exit the spinal canal.

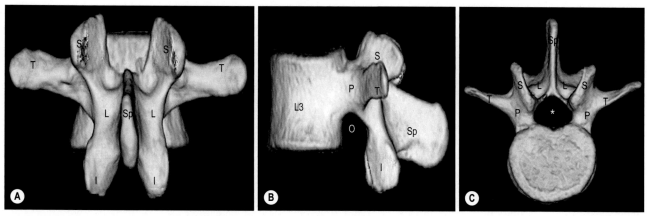

FIGURE 1-3 ■ **Normal imaging anatomy of the lumbar spine on CT.** 3D reformatted CT images of L3 in posterior (A), lateral (B) and superior (C) views. P = pedicle, L = lamina, I = inferior articular process, S = superior articular process, Sp = spinous process, T = transverse process, O = intervertebral foramen, * = spinal canal.

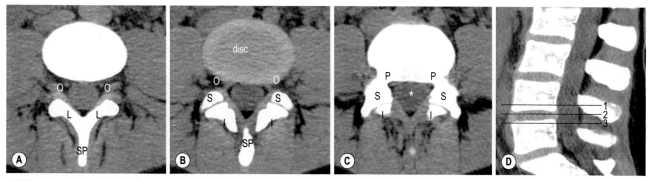

FIGURE 1-4 ■ **Normal imaging anatomy of the posterior arch of the lumbar spine on CT.** Axial images (A, B, C) at different levels as indicated on the sagittal (D) image. P = pedicle, L = lamina, I = inferior articular process, S = superior articular process, Sp = spinous process, T = transverse process, O = intervertebral foramen, * = spinal canal.

Spinous and Transverse Processes

The spinous process is attached to the most posterior part of the neural arch. The transverse processes arise from the lateral edge of each neural arch (Figs. 1-2–1-4). The spinous as well as the transverse process serve as an important site of attachment for the deep back muscles. As described above, they also divide the neural arch into different anatomical parts.

JOINTS

Facet Joints

The facet joints or the zygapophyseal joints are diarthrodial synovial joints between the inferior and superior articular processes of adjacent neural arches. These articular processes arise from the articular pillars including the bone at the junction between pedicles and the laminae. The superior articular process is located relative anterior to the inferior articular process and faces posteriorly (Figs. 1-2–1-4). In the lumbar spine the joint surface is located in an oblique way at an angle of about

45° between the sagittal and coronal plane. In the thoracic spine the facet joints are almost orientated in the coronal plan.[5]

The inferior facets have a convex shape while the superior articular surface has a concave aspect. In a non-degenerative spine the joint surface is covered with hyaline cartilage, being the thickest in the centre of the joint. In the normal anatomy, as most other joints, the surface of the joints should be smooth and regular with an equal spacing between the two joint surfaces. The distance between the articular processes at the facet joint should be between 2 and 4 mm on plain radiography.[6]

On the posterolateral side, the facet joint is covered with a strong fibrous capsule which is composed of several layers of fibrous tissue and a synovial membrane. On the anterior side of the joint, there is no fibrous capsule. Here, the only border between the spinal canal and the facet joint is formed by the ligamentum flavum and the synovial membrane.[7] The capsule is composed of a superior and inferior recess containing fat pads. These fat pads act as movement-compensating mechanisms and as a lubrication mechanism for the facet joint as they are partially covered with synovial tissue.[5]

Intervertebral Disc—Symphysis

The intervertebral disc consists of the inner nucleus pulposus surrounded by an outer layer, the annulus fibrosus. Embryologically the nucleus pulposus is formed from cells originating from the notochord; in humans these notochordial cells are lost and replaced by chondrocyte-like cells. The nucleus pulposus is macroscopically composed of soft, elastic tissue with a yellow colour.[8] The nucleus pulposus is primarily composed of water, proteoglycans and loose collagen fibres. With normal ageing the water content decreases.

The outer annulus fibrosus is composed of multiple concentric layers of fibrocartilage tissue. The outer layers, also called Sharpey's fibres, continue in the longitudinal ligament and the vertebral bodies. The fibres of each layer are directed in an oblique way (30° angle), forming a meshwork. In this way a very strong flexible structure is formed.

LIGAMENTS

Longitudinal Ligaments

A longitudinal ligament is present at the anterior and posterior part of the vertebral bodies running along the entire spine, providing stability (Fig. 1-5). The anterior longitudinal ligament (ALL) is a thick ligament which is slightly thinner at the level of the vertebral bodies and wider at the intervertebral disc.

The posterior longitudinal ligament (PLL) is situated in the vertebral canal and runs from the dens axis (tectorial membrane) to the sacrum. It is thicker in the thoracic spine and wider in the cervical region compared to the lumbar level. At the level of the vertebral bodies the PLL is separated from the concave posterior wall of the vertebral bodies by the anterior epidural space. This space contains epidural fat, basivertebral veins and the anterior internal vertebral veins.

Ligamentum Flavum

The ligamentum flavum or yellow ligament is a paired structure connecting the spinal laminae forming the posterior wall of the spinal canal (Fig. 1-6). At the lateral side these structures fuse with the capsule of the facet joints, forming a boundary of the intervertebral neuroforamina.[9] The boundary between the two ligamenta flava in the centre is indistinguishable on imaging. The ligamenta flava provide a static elastic force to stimulate the return to a neutral position after flexion or extension. They also limit the flexion motion of the spine and help maintain a smooth posterior lining of the central spinal canal.[10]

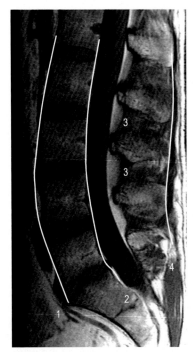

FIGURE 1-5 ■ **Normal anatomy of the spinal ligaments.** Sagittal T$_1$-weighted MRI image of the lumbar spine. 1 = anterior longitudinal ligament, 2 = posterior longitudinal ligament, 3 = interspinous ligament, 4 = supraspinous ligament.

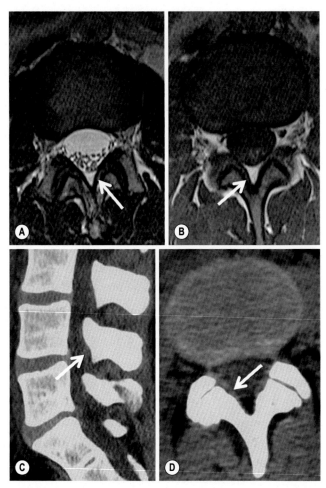

FIGURE 1-6 ■ **Ligamentum flavum.** Axial T$_1$-weighted (A) and T$_2$-weighted (B) images; sagittal (C) and axial (D) reformatted CT images. The ligamentum flavum or yellow ligament (indicated with arrow) is a thin ligament connecting the laminae and forms the posterior wall of the spinal canal.

Interconnecting Ligaments

The posterior elements are heavily reinforced with different ligaments connecting two adjacent vertebra. The supraspinous ligament connects the tips from the spinous processes while the interspinous ligaments connect the base of the adjacent spinous processes (Fig. 1-5). The transverse processes are connected by the intertransverse ligaments. As discussed earlier the laminae of the adjacent vertebra are bound together by the ligamentum flavum.

NEURAL STRUCTURES—SPINAL CORD, SPINAL NERVES, DURA MATER

The shape of the spinal canal varies from oval on the cervical and thoracic level to a triangular shape at the lower lumbar region.[11]

Anteriorly the dura mater is in contact with the posterior longitudinal ligament almost over the length of the whole spine. Laterally the dura mater is in close contact with the medial border of the pedicles. Above and below the pedicles the dura mater is in contact with the epidural fat in continuity with the intervertebral foramina. Posteriorly the dura mater is in contact with the posterior epidural fat separating the dura from the ligamenta flava, the posterior joints and the laminae.

In the kyphotic thoracic regions, the dura can be separated from the posterior elements by a layer of epidural fat of up to 5 mm thick. This fat should not be mistaken for epidural lipomatosis.

The spinal cord and its normal internal structure (grey and white matter) are best evaluated with MR imaging (T_2). It consists of a central butterfly-shaped part which is the grey matter. The measurements of the spinal cord show a wide variation according to the patient.

The conus medullaris is the terminal end of the spinal cord and is in normal anatomy found at the level L1–L2. The spinal cord tapers out into a cone at this level and the nerve roots descend, forming the cauda equina.

The spinal nerves exit the spinal canal through the intervertebral neuroforamina. At the cervical and thoracic level the nerve roots leave the spinal canal horizontally. At the lumbar level the nerve roots first descend in the lateral canal recess before exiting through the neuroforamen.

VASCULAR STRUCTURES

The spinal cord is supplied by three main arteries parallel to the spinal cord: one anterior and two posterior. The blood supply can be divided into three anatomical regions. In the cervicothoracic region the blood is supplied segmentally from arteries originating from the vertebral arteries and the great vessels of the neck (i.e. aorta, carotid and subclavian arteries). The midthoracic region receives most of its blood supply from collateral circulation from superior and inferior arteries and acts as a watershed area. The segmental blood supply is received from small perforants originating from the aorta. The thoracolumbar region is supplied by segmental arteries from the aorta and the iliac arteries. Variably originating from levels Th9 to L2 and in most cases from the left side of the vertebral column, the largest vessel originates from the aorta: the artery of Adamkiewicz.

The venous plexus in the spine is called the Batson plexus. This plexus is unique compared to other plexuses in the body as this venous plexus does not have valves, allowing retrograde flow in the venous network.

CRANIOCERVICAL JUNCTION

The craniocervical junction (CCJ) is the region connecting a spherical (head) and a tubular structure (spine). To stabilise this connection the craniocervical junction is composed of bones, ligaments and muscles.

The bony parts are formed by the occipital bone with a basilar part, squamous part (scale) and the lateral (condylar) part. At the cervical part of the connection, the atlas (C1) consists of an anterior and posterior arch, and two bulky lateral masses. The axis (C2) is formed by a vertebral body, pedicles, foramina transversaria, laminae, spinous process and the dens axis articulating anteriorly with the arcus anterior of the atlas.

The complex organisation of ligaments at the CCJ provides stability but allows a complex range of motion. These ligaments can be divided into the external and internal ligaments. The anterior external ligaments are formed by the ALL running along the anterior side of the vertebral bodies from C2 downward and the anterior atlanto-axial ligament connecting the ALL and the arcus anterior of the atlas. The ligament running between the arcus anterior of the atlas and the os occipitale is the atlanto-occipital ligament. Posteriorly the external ligaments consist of the extension of the ligamenta flava, the posterior atlanto-occipital and the posterior atlanto-axial ligament. The ligamentum nuchae runs from the external occipital protuberance to the spinous process of C7.

The internal ligaments of the CCJ consist anteriorly of a thin apical ligament and thick alar ligaments. The alar ligaments attach the axis to the skull base and run from the lateral aspect of the odontoid process to the anterior part of the foramen magnum. The middle internal ligament (cruciform ligament) is formed by the transverse ligament of C1, the accessory ligaments and the superior and inferior fibres. The transverse ligament is the largest, strongest and thickest craniocervical ligament and maintains stability by locking the anterior part of the odontoid process against the posterior side of the anterior arch of the atlas.[12] It runs posterior to the odontoid process of the dens and attaches bilaterally on the lateral tubercle of C1. The posterior internal ligament is the tectorial membrane. Superiorly this ligament continues as the dura mater; inferiorly the ligament forms the posterior longitudinal ligament.

The function of the muscles in the CCJ is to initiate and maintain movement, and not to limit the movements of this joint. They can be grouped into flexion, extension, abduction, adduction and rotation.

IMAGING TECHNIQUES

Multiple imaging techniques are available to evaluate the spine. The choice of imaging technique depends on the indication (e.g. traumatic or non-traumatic) and on the age of the patient. As MRI has become widely available in most countries it has become the first examination to perform in a non-traumatic setting. Especially in young patients it has the advantage not to use X-rays. In older patients computed tomography can be indicated to evaluate bony degenerative changes. If a contraindication for MRI is present, other imaging techniques (e.g. CT) are indicated.

In post-traumatic imaging CT is the preferred initial imaging technique in blunt spinal trauma patients. CT is also indicated in acute trauma patients when there is no optimal visualisation of the spine on plain film and in patients with unexplained focal pain or neurological deficit with a negative plain film, if unexplained soft-tissue swelling is present or when plain film is abnormal. Plain radiography can be performed in minor injuries. CT offers outstanding information about the bony lesions of the spine and reconstruction in virtually every anatomical plane. A group at the Harborview Medical Center in Seattle, Washington, defined a series of high-risk criteria to decide whether to perform plain radiography or CT imaging as the primary technique when imaging cervical spinal trauma (Table 1-1).[13]

In the evaluation of low back pain (LBP) with or without radiculopathy careful selection of the patients to undergo imaging is indicated to work cost-effectively. Uncomplicated acute (less than 6 weeks) LBP and/or radiculopathy is often self-limiting and imaging is not indicated. Imaging should be considered if any 'red flags' (Table 1-2) are present or if complaints show no

TABLE 1-1 Harborview High-Risk Criteria

If yes to any criteria, high risk for c-spine injury and indication for CT
- Presence of significant head injury
- Presence of focal neurological deficit(s)
- Presence of pelvic or multiple extremity fractures
- Combined impact of accident >50 km/h (>35 mph)
- Death at the scene of the motor vehicle accident
- Accident involved a fall from a height of 3 m or more

TABLE 1-2 'Red Flags' in Low Back Pain

- Trauma, cumulative trauma
- Unexplained weight loss, insidious onset
- Age >50 years with osteoporosis or compression fractures
- Unexplained fever, history of urinary or other infection
- Immunosuppression, diabetes mellitus
- History of cancer
- Intravenous drug use
- Prolonged use of corticosteroids, osteoporosis
- Age >70 years
- Focal neurological deficit(s) with progressive or disabling symptoms, cauda equina syndrome
- Duration longer than 6 weeks
- Prior surgery

improvement after 6 weeks.[14] Plain radiography can be useful in all of the conditions noted in Table 1-2 but can be sufficient if normal in patients with recent significant trauma or osteoporosis or age >70 years. In patients with LBP complicated with red flags, MRI or CT can be justified. MRI is the examination of choice, while CT should be considered in patients with contraindications for MRI or in postoperative patients.

PLAIN RADIOGRAPHY

Conventional X-ray imaging is a fast, easy and inexpensive technique which offers a good overview of a large segment of the spine. It is still widely used, but cannot be justified any longer as the definite examination. Plain radiography still has the advantage over CT and MRI for the evaluation of structural malformations and instability with or without dynamic imaging in erect position.

The main disadvantage of plain radiographs is the superimposition of soft tissue and bony structures, making the interpretation difficult. In the lateral view the cervicothoracic junction can be difficult to visualise due to superimposition of the shoulders. To overcome this problem a so-called swimmer's view is made by elevating one arm above the head and letting the other hang down by the side. At the thoracolumbar junction the diaphragm makes it difficult to interpret the lateral view. On the anteroposterior (AP) view superimposition of heart and mediastinum in the thoracic spine and bowel structures in the lumbar spine offer evaluation difficulties.

In a post-traumatic setting, plain radiography can be used to determine the level of the injury to perform a CT of only one specific region. In the cervical spine, studies show that up to 55% of clinically significant fractures can be missed on plain radiography.[15]

In the cervical spine AP and lateral views are the standard views of the cervical spine. To make a good assessment of the spine, a high-quality image with visualisation of the seven cervical vertebral bodies as well as the first thoracic vertebra is necessary (Fig. 1-7). The lateral view is considered the most important view as 90% of pathology can be seen in this image. To evaluate the dens and the atlanto-axial joints an AP 'transbuccal' view is essential (Fig. 1-8). In post-traumatic patients with neck collars, this view can be difficult to perform and if there is any doubt a CT examination should be performed. Oblique views are performed to evaluate the neuroforamina. Two views are taken with the patient turned 45° to either side. The neuroforamen viewed en face is the contralateral side to which the patient has turned the head. The need for these views can be questioned as MRI and especially CT offers a much better evaluation of the (bony) neuroforamina and may demonstrate nerve root compression.

In the thoracic spine, an AP and lateral view is performed. The AP view is used to assess the pedicles (possible metastasis) and the vertebral alignment (scoliosis). When performing the lateral view the convexity of a possible scoliosis should be turned towards the film so the

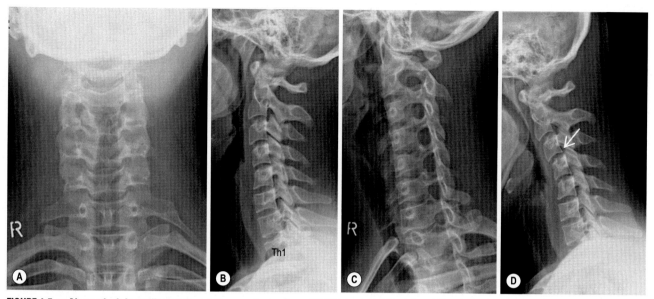

FIGURE 1-7 ■ **Normal plain radiography of the cervical spine.** AP (A), lateral (B), right oblique (C) and dynamic flexion (D) views of the cervical spine. Decreased cervical lordosis of the cervical spine (B) due to erect positioning of the patient; the upper part of Th1 (Th1) is visualised as it should. In the right oblique (C) there is no obliteration of the left intervertebral neuroforamina. On the dynamic flexion (D) we see a decreased mobility of the lower vertebral segments; the minimal anterolisthesis (arrow) as seen at C3–C4 is normal during flexion.

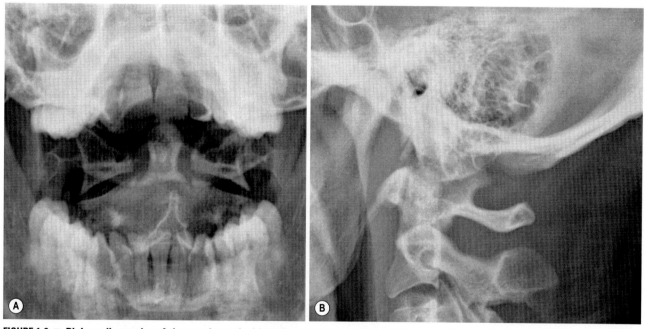

FIGURE 1-8 ■ **Plain radiography of the craniocervical junction.** AP (A) and lateral (B) views of the craniocervical junction. A complete free projection of the dens should be obtained, although sometimes difficult in post-traumatic patients. In this case the patient's head is turned slightly to the right, causing a discrete asymmetric position of the dens within the atlas. (Note the plumb line between teeth 11 and 21 doesn't project through the centre of the dens.)

divergent X-rays are more parallel to the disc spaces. Autotomography (the patient breaths gently during exposure) is used to blur out the ribs and diaphragm.

In the lumbar spine, the posteroanterior (PA) image of the lumbar spine is taken from posterior to anterior as the divergent X-ray beam will be more parallel to the disc spaces (Fig. 1-9) and to lessen radiation to the organs. When taken from anterior to posterior, flexion of hips and knees will reduce the lumbar lordosis. A spot image of the L5–S1 disc space is made from anterior to posterior with a caudocranial inclination of the tube. The hips and knees are in flexion to reduce the lumbar lordosis. As

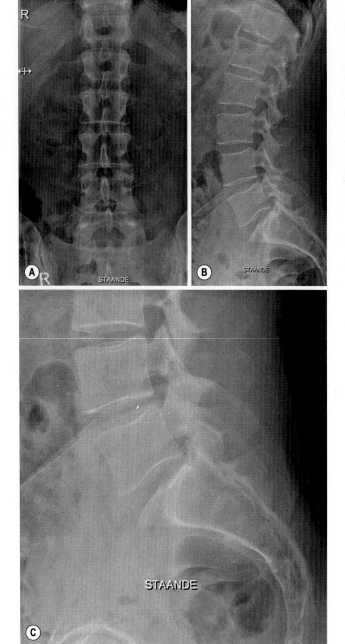

FIGURE 1-9 ■ **Normal plain radiography of the lumbar spine.** PA (A), lateral (B) and lateral spot S1 (C) views. The spot image of L5–S1 is taken anteroposteriorly with the X-ray beam parallel to the intervertebral disc space.

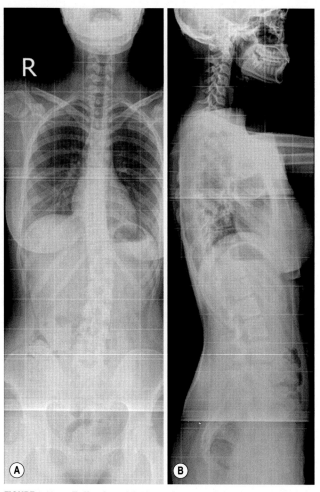

FIGURE 1-10 ■ **Full spine.** AP (A) and lateral (B) views of full spine in erect position. The AP view (A) shows a sinistroconvex scoliosis of the lumbar spine. The plumb line through the centre of C7 projects < 2 cm lateral of the plumb line through the centre of the sacrum, indicating a compensated scoliosis. The lateral view (B) shows a normal thoracic kyphosis and lumbar lordosis.

in the thoracic spine, the convexity of a scoliosis, if present, should be nearer to the radiograph. The PA oblique view is acquired by turning the patient 45°; a torsion of the lumbar spine should be avoided. The oblique view of the lumbar spine is especially useful for evaluating the facet joints and pedicles; this can be used in identification of a spondylolisthesis.

A full-spine AP view is used to evaluate and measure scoliosis and anatomical anomalies of the spine

(Fig. 1-10). The lateral view is used to evaluate the thoracic kyphosis and lumbar and cervical lordosis.

Functional (extension/flexion) lateral views can be made to evaluate instability. On these images it is important to look for displacement of the vertebral bodies (anterolisthesis or retrolisthesis) or increased displacement of the vertebral bodies and an increase in distance between the spinous process (Fig. 1-7). In the lumbar spine this is often performed in patients with spondylolisthesis or after surgery to evaluate instability.

MYELOGRAPHY

Myelography and post-myelography computed tomography (Fig. 1-11) for the evaluation of spinal pathology have been largely replaced by MR imaging. MR imaging has the advantage of being non-invasive, painless and without X-ray irradiation and offers multiplanar imaging

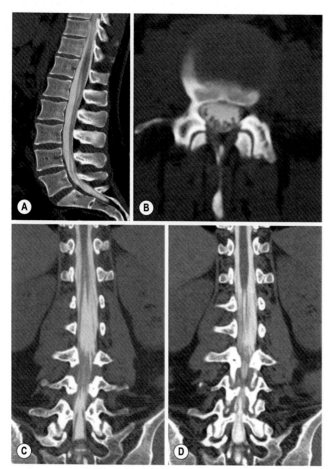

FIGURE 1-11 ■ **Post-myelography CT examination.** Sagittal (A), axial (B) and curved coronal (C, D) reformatted CT images after myelography. Normal imaging study of the spinal canal in a patient with MR-incompatible implants shows the position of the nerve roots of the cauda equina in the spinal canal as well as possible spinal canal stenosis.

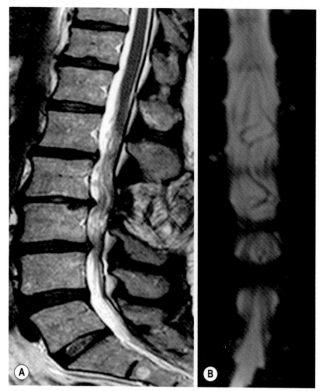

FIGURE 1-12 ■ **MR-myelography.** T_2-weighted (A) and MR myelography (B) images. Postoperative status after laminectomy at L2–L3 for a spinal canal stenosis. Sagittal T_2-weighted image and the myelo-MR show residual redundant nerve roots of the cauda equina proximal to the previous spinal canal stenosis.

possibilities. Therefore an important clinical indication is necessary to perform myelography. Myelographic MR images are obtained without the injection of intrathecal contrast and can be useful for evaluating the spinal canal (Fig. 1-12). The downside is a lower signal-to-noise ratio (SNR) of MR compared to X-ray myelography; thus small lesions can be missed on myelographic MR images.[16]

At this moment only a few indications remain for myelography; contraindications for the patient to undergo MR examinations (e.g. non-compatible pacemaker) are severe claustrophobia or absence of MR imaging. X-ray myelography can be used to dynamically evaluate the spinal canal in patients with spondylolisthesis. Myelography can be used to evaluate processes contacting, impinging or displacing the thecal sac or the nerve roots (e.g. arachnoiditis). Myelography has the advantage over MRI of allowing dynamic and functional evaluation of the cerebrospinal fluid (CSF) and the evaluation of active CSF leakage. Myelography can also be useful in a postoperative spine where artefacts of surgical material may obscure the spinal canal or nerve roots on MRI.[17]

Before starting the examination, patients should be screened. Patients with prior allergic reactions to contrast media should be premedicated. Because intrathecal iodinated contrast medium carries a risk of seizures, medication that provokes seizures should be stopped 48 hours before until 24 hours after the examination. The patients' international normalised ratio (INR) should be normal and ideally less than 1.5 and all woman of childbearing age should be screened for pregnancy.

For myelography a 22- to 26-gauge needle may be used; the smaller the bore, the smaller the risk for CSF leakage after the procedure. Typically a Quincke-type needle with a sharp tip is used for easy penetration of the skin and optimal steering of the needle. A non-ionic contrast agent proved for intrathecal use should be used to reduce neurotoxicity.

The patient is placed in a prone position with the hand above the head and his left knee up providing stability and an oblique view to open the interlaminar spaces. Using fluoroscopy, the level L2–L3 is localised. The region is disinfected and locally anaesthetised. A lumbar puncture is performed and the subarachnoidal location controlled. A test injection with 1–2 mL of contrast medium is performed under fluoroscopy and a 'wisp of smoke' appearance indicates free flow and subarachnoidal placement.

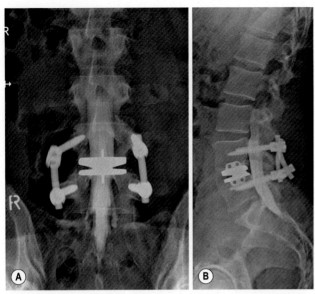

FIGURE 1-13 ■ **Plain film myelography.** AP (A) and lateral (B) plain film images after myelography in a postoperative patient who had a posterior lumbar intervertebral fusion (PLIF) and disc prosthesis at L4–L5. Myelography shows no spinal canal stenosis.

For lumbar myelography the patient is tilted with the feet down (reverse Trendelenburg) , causing the contrast medium to pool in the thecal sac. AP and oblique views as well as lateral views are performed (Fig. 1-13). The left lateral decubitus is performed as it is easier for the radiologist to position the patient. With the patient in lateral decubitus the table is put flat to take a lateral view of the thoracolumbar junction.[17] The thoracic and cervical myelography is seldom performed and should be done by an experienced radiologist. In most cases a lumbar contrast injection is performed and the table is placed in Trendelenburg position to allow contrast medium to flow to the thoracic and cervical level.

SPINAL ANGIOGRAPHY

Imaging of the vascular structures of the spine is challenging because of the very small vessels, variable and complex anatomy with multiple feeders at different levels. A technique with a high spatial resolution is needed for reliable and accurate visualisation.[18] For this reason digital subtraction angiography (DSA) still remains the gold standard. In clinical practice, however, computed tomographic angiography (CTA) or MR angiography (MRA) can be used to visualise the vascular malformation and the level of vascular feeders. In this way, DSA can be focused on a selection of supplying blood vessels, and examination time, contrast and radiation dose are reduced. A study of 15 patients by Nijenhuis et al. showed that the level of the Adamkiewicz artery can be sufficiently visualised with contrast-enhanced MRA in 14 out of 15 patients, although DSA still offers superior imaging

quality.[19] For the evaluation of the spinal arteries on CTA, a high injection rate of 6 mL/s with a high concentration contrast agent is needed to show the spinal cord vessels.[18]

Indications for spinal angiography are suspicion of arteriovenous (AV) malformations, spinal aneurysms, vascular tumours of the spinal cord, meninges or vertebral column (Fig. 1-14). It can also be used for preoperative visualisation of the Adamkiewicz artery in cases of aorta or spinal surgery.[20] On MR imaging, small flow artefacts can simulate a vascular malformation. Thin slices and imaging after gadolinium can be used to differentiate between a flow artefact and a vascular malformation and to avoid spinal DSA.

As spinal DSA is a complex, invasive investigation with risk of morbidity it should only be performed in an experienced centre. Because catheter spinal angiography is an invasive, time-consuming procedure with risk of morbidity and a relative high cost the results of this examination should have a benefit or therapeutical implication for the patient. An intervention with embolisation is also possible when performing spinal angiography.

COMPUTED TOMOGRAPHY

Computed tomography of the spine is the first choice of examination in trauma patients with a high sensitivity in detecting fractures. Although MRI has become more common for the evaluation of the disc space and the spinal canal, CT is still adequate enough to visualise the spinal cord, exclude compression (e.g. haematoma or disc herniation) and is very useful in evaluating the posterior elements and bony changes as facet joint pathology and Baastrup's phenomenon. After surgery, CT can visualise the surgical materials and evaluate possible loosening.

The patient is placed in supine position on the CT table with the neck gently flexed (in non-traumatic patients) to reduce the cervical lordosis. Modern spiral CT allows a fast and continuous acquisition of data to obtain a full data set which makes reconstructions in all anatomical planes as well as 3D reconstruction possible (Fig. 1-15). A digital radiograph, also known as a 'scout' image or 'localiser' (lateral, AP view or both), of the region of interest is performed to make a selection of the volume to be imaged. This scout film can retrospectively be used to localise the level of the acquired data. During examination of the spine it is not necessary to do a breath-hold command.

After the acquisition of the data reconstructions in the sagittal and axial (parallel to the vertebral discs) planes are performed, the slice thickness depends on the region of interest and the indication of the examination. A soft-tissue and bone algorithm is used to enable evaluation of the bone (high resolution of bone structures) and soft tissue. The multislice volume imaging allows reconstructions in virtually every plane as well as curved reconstructions in patients with scoliosis. Three-dimensional volumetric reconstructions can be made to make illustrative images for the clinicians.

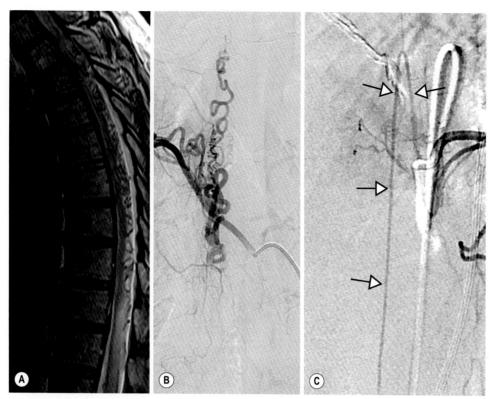

FIGURE 1-14 ■ Sagittal T_2-weighted image (A) of the thoracic spine and selective DSA of the right lumbar artery Th6 (B) and of the left lumbar artery Th8 (C). (A) An AV malformation posterior of the myelum with a high signal intensity in the myelum indicating myelomalacia. (B) The AV malformation selective contrast injection in the right lumbar artery at the level Th6. (C) The Adamkiewicz artery (arrow), with its origin at the left lumbar artery at Th8.

MAGNETIC RESONANCE IMAGING

Magnetic resonance imaging has become the method of choice for imaging of the spine. It is a non-invasive technique and is not associated with radiation exposure. As the signal intensity of CSF, bone, disc, spinal cord and epidural fat are different on most sequences, the contrast resolution can be decreased, which improves the spatial resolution.

The specific parameters of the sequences, the coil type and the reduction of motion artefacts are dependent on the individual manufacturers; the general principles are, however, the same.

The MRI examination starts with acquiring a coronal, low-resolution multislice sequence as a localiser. On these images the most optimal sagittal plane is chosen to make high-resolution images of the spine. A spatial pre-saturation slab is applied in the cervical spine over the larynx and the carotid artery. In the thoracic spine the same technique is used to reduce artefacts from heart and aorta. The axial images are planned on the high-resolution sagittal images over the regions of interest.

We suggest using sagittal T_1, sagittal T_2, sagittal T_2 with fat suppression (e.g. STIR) and axial T_2 as a routine protocol in MRI of the spine. In the lumbar spine we routinely add axial T_1. According to the clinical information, additional sequences can be added as required.

In the postoperative lumbar spine, again, the routine protocol is used. In addition, sagittal and axial T_1-weighted images after gadolinium (Gd) are acquired.

Spin-Echo T_1-Weighted Imaging

An MR image is called a 'T1-weighted' image when image contrast is based upon difference in longitudinal relaxation time (T_1). T_1 is a time constant specific for each tissue and is characterised by the rate in which the longitudinal magnetisation is restored. T_1 is traditionally produced using spin-echo (SE) sequences with a short repetition time (TR 300–700 ms) and short echo time (TE < 30 ms). If a SE sequence is used with a short TR, spins with a long T_1 relaxation time cannot completely relax and do not contribute to the signal.

In T_1 these tissues (e.g. CSF) are seen as dark structures. Tissues with a short T_1 relaxation time (e.g. fat) conversely have a high signal intensity. T_1-weighted images provide excellent anatomical detail, including bone marrow changes, osseous structures, discs and soft tissue.[21]

Contrast-Enhanced T_1-Weighted Imaging

Contrast agents used in MR imaging contain ions with a high electron spin, causing a shortening of relaxation

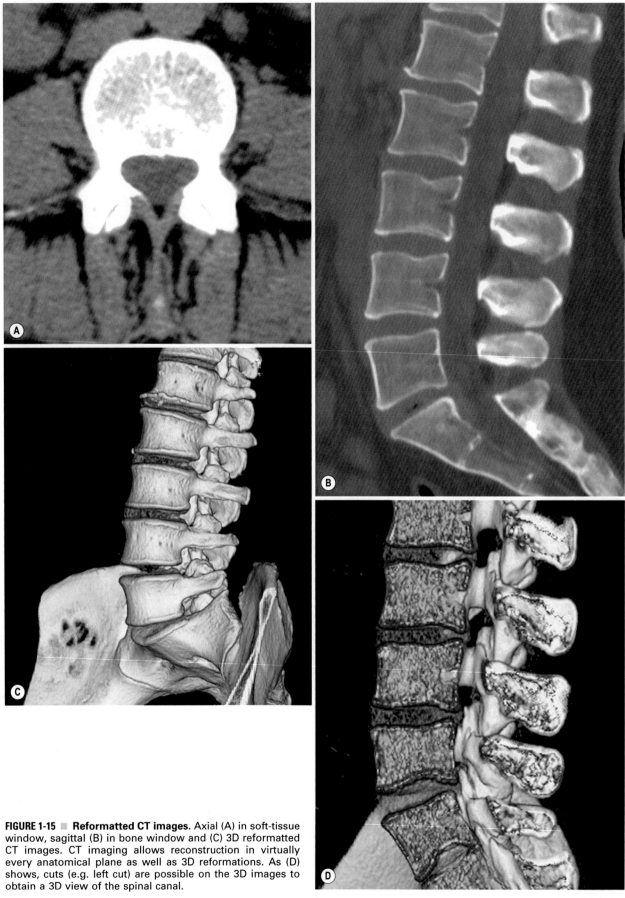

FIGURE 1-15 ■ **Reformatted CT images.** Axial (A) in soft-tissue window, sagittal (B) in bone window and (C) 3D reformatted CT images. CT imaging allows reconstruction in virtually every anatomical plane as well as 3D reformations. As (D) shows, cuts (e.g. left cut) are possible on the 3D images to obtain a 3D view of the spinal canal.

time in adjacent molecules in a magnetic field. The paramagnetic contrast agents for intravenous injection are gadolinium chelates. The standard dose for intravenous injected gadolinium is 0.1 mmol/kg body weight. Gadolinium-based paramagnetic contrast agents are relatively safe and seldom give allergic reactions.[22] Enhancement after injection of paramagnetic contrast agents is seen as an increase in signal intensity and is best seen on T_1. Gadolinium chelates not only shorten T_1 but also T_2. For the evaluation of enhancement it is recommended to perform pre- and post-contrast images over the same region (Fig. 1-16).

The enhancement mechanism is different between intra- and extra-axial lesions. In intra-axial lesions enhancement is caused by disruption of the blood–brain barrier, whereas in extra-axial lesions it is caused by hypervascularity.

Post-contrast imaging can be used to distinguish post-operative fibrosis (scarring) from recurrent disc fragments.[23] In the lumbar spine, fat-suppression techniques before and/or after contrast-enhanced T_1 can further assist in differentiating between enhancing scar tissue and epidural fat and, in rare cases, between postoperative blood and normal epidural fat.[24]

Fat suppression on T_1-weighted images before intravenous injection of gadolinium is of little value because the signal from most pathological lesions, whether inflammatory, neoplastic or infectious, is often low and better visualised against the bright signal intensity of fat. In post-gadolinium T_1-weighted fat suppression can be useful in adults with fatty transformation of the bone marrow. Fat-suppressed images can be particularly useful for evaluating ligamentous structures or lesions involving the paraspinal tissues.[21]

Spin-Echo and Fast Spin-Echo T_2-Weighted Imaging

An MR image is called a 'T_2-weighted' image when image contrast is based upon the difference in transverse relaxation time (T_2 time). In SE sequences, T_2 weighting is achieved by applying a long repetition time (TR 2000–3000 ms) and a long echo time (TE 80–120 ms). T_1 is thus reduced by the long TR while the T_2 contrast is strong due to the long TE. The long TR time imposes a high acquisition time, which is a disadvantage for the conventional SE sequences.

In fast spin-echo (FSE) sequences (also called turbo spin-echo or TSE), multiple phase-encoding steps are acquired per excitation instead of a single step as in conventional SE sequences, causing a reduction in acquiring time.

Imaging characteristics of SE and FSE T_2 are comparable. Fat (including fatty bone marrow), however, is brighter on FSE than on SE sequences; this may mask vertebral metastasis on FSE T_2.

Bright CSF is the hallmark of T_2-weighted images. The spinal cord and nerves have an intermediate signal intensity, causing a maximal contrast between the CSF and neural tissue[21] (Fig. 1-17). T_2-weighted images have

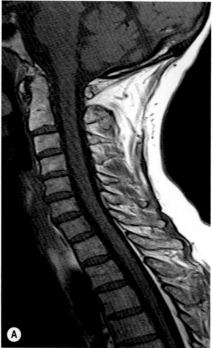
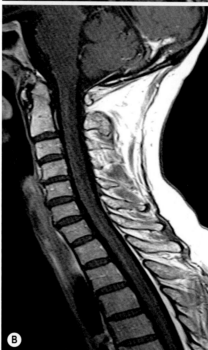

FIGURE 1-16 ■ Sagittal T_1-weighted images before (A) and after (B) injection of gadolinium. The normal enhancement of vascular structures post-contrast indicates the presence of contrast as seen posterior of C2 in and in de venous sinus.

a high sensitivity in detecting pathological changes in tissue, especially in which the extracellular matrix has a higher water content.

Gradient-Echo Imaging

Gradient-recalled echo (GRE) images appear to be SE or FSE T_2-weighted, as CSF has a high signal intensity; the

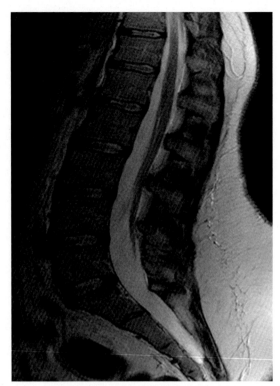

FIGURE 1-17 ▪ **T$_2$-weighted image of the lumbar spine.** Normal sagittal T$_2$-weighted image of the lumbar spine. On T$_2$-weighted images there is a maximal contrast between the cerebrospinal fluid and the spinal cord and nerves.

intervertebral discs have a relatively high signal intensity and the vertebrae a low signal. Blood flow creates a high signal intensity on these images.

GRE T$_2$* has the advantage over conventional SE sequences of offering shorter echo times and, as such, less CSF-pulsation artefacts are especially useful in the cervical and thoracic spine.

A disadvantage of GRE is the low contrast for intramedullary lesions compared with SE or FSE. The signal-to-noise is superior in FSE imaging sequences compared with GRE. GRE images are also more susceptible to local field inhomogeneity of the magnetic field and signal loss is exaggerated in the presence of these inhomogeneities, e.g. metallic implants.

Short Tau Inversion Recovery

Short tau inversion recovery (STIR) has a high sensitivity in detecting musculoskeletal disease because of the synergistic effect of prolonged T$_1$ and T$_2$ in abnormal tissue, with improved SNR and fat suppression[25] (Fig. 1-18). This technique is especially favourable in detecting degenerative changes (Modic-changes, facet joint degeneration, spondylolysis, Baastrup) and vertebral metastasis. STIR (and fast-STIR) has also proved to be useful in detecting MS lesions compared with T$_2$-weighted images.

Because of the longer acquisition time, this technique is more prone to motion artefacts and is not indicated

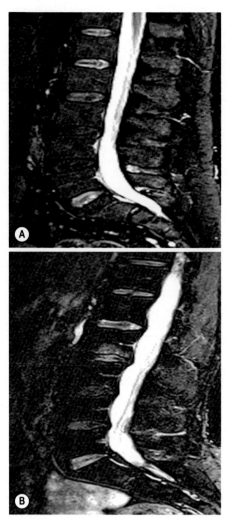

FIGURE 1-18 ▪ **Sagittal STIR images** of the lumbar spine in a patient with a normal STIR image (A) with TR 4510 and TE 63. (B) Increased signal intensity on the STIR image (TR 3210, TE 52) in the lower endplate of L2, indicating oedema.

for evaluation of the thoracic spine.[26] STIR images tend to be noisy, but the usefulness is provided by the high SNR.

Diffusion-Weighted Imaging

Diffusion-weighted imaging (DWI) and the calculated apparent diffusion coefficient (ADC) maps are widely used for evaluating many diseases in the brain (Fig. 1-19). In the spine and the vertebral column the research on DWI is much more limited and poses some difficulties, due to the higher magnetic inhomogeneities in and around the spine such as the smaller size, the low SNR and the involuntary motion (respiration and vascular motion). DWI on the spinal cord can be adopted to evaluate spinal cord infarction, active MS lesions, spinal compression and post-traumatic injury. DWI can also be used to detect drop metastasis in children with hypercellular brain tumours.[27] In addition, although still in

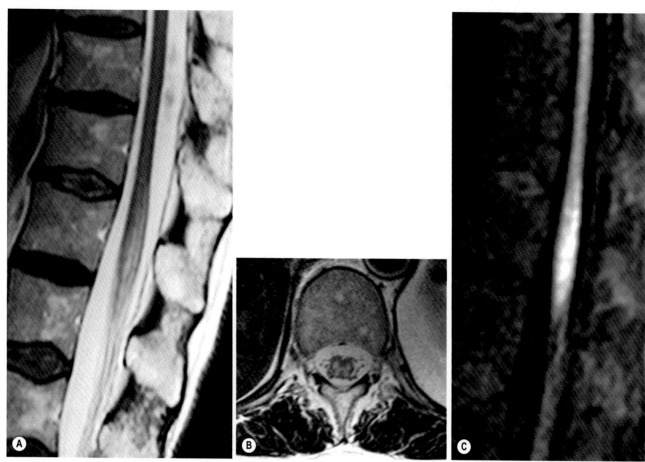

FIGURE 1-19 ■ **Diffusion-weighted imaging: sagittal (A) and axial (B) T₂-weighted and (C) sagittal diffusion-weighted images.** (A) Oedema of the distal and of the spinal cord with hyperintense signal intensity. (B) A hyperintense signal centrally in the grey matter, also known as the 'owl's eye'. The diffusion-weighted image (C) shows diffusion restriction in the distal spinal cord, indicating ischaemia (Images courtesy of Prof. Dr. M. Thurnher, Vienna Austria).

research, diffusion tensor imaging (DTI) can be used to allow characterisation of the structural integrity of the spinal cord.

Fluid-Attenuated Inversion Recovery

The primary goal of fluid-attenuated inversion recovery (FLAIR) sequences is to improve contrast in cases where resolution is less important. FLAIR is a highly T₂-weighted SE sequence with a long inversion recovery time suppressing all the signal from the CSF (black on FLAIR). In the spine this removes the motion artefacts from the CSF.

In FLAIR images most lesions have a high signal intensity; however, cystic lesions and cysts will also appear as black areas (signal voids). In imaging of the lumbar spine on 3 T some studies suggest T₁-weighted FLAIR images to be superior in delineating normal tissue interfaces between soft tissue/CSF-bone or disc/CSF compared with T₁-weighted FSE technique.[28]

Three-Dimensional (3D) Imaging

Volume or 3D imaging is a technique of acquiring thin slices without a reduced SNR or increase in imaging time. GRE and FSE sequences can be used to obtain a 3D data set. When using 3D GRE imaging, a short TR is preferred because of the large number of phase-encoding pulses required. This sequence is vulnerable to motion-induced phase shifts.

An FSE sequence with thin (1–2 mm) slices can be used to cover a segment of the spine. Three-dimensional FSE offers the advantage of reducing flow void artefacts in the CSF.

A 3D data set with thin slices can be used to make reconstructions in multiple imaging planes by using multiplanar reformatting algorithms.

Artefacts

Artefacts are defined as any images (signal or signal loss) that have no anatomical basis but are the result of distorted, additional or suppressed information. Many artefacts are caused by poor choice of technical parameters or defective MRI unit. For example, 3 T compared with 1.5 T MRI gives more artefacts; they are both increased in size as well as in numbers. A good knowledge of normal anatomy and pathology will improve detection of these artefacts.

Susceptibility Artefacts

Magnetic susceptibility artefacts occur at the boundary of two tissues with a large difference in magnetic susceptibility, e.g. the presence of ferromagnetic materials or an air–tissue interface. In the spine this kind of artefact is caused by the presence of metal implants as seen in the postoperative spine and results from a vast difference in magnetic properties between metal implants and human tissue. The sensitivity of the different pulse sequences to these artefacts is echoplanar (EPI) > gradient echo (GRE) > spin echo (SE) > fast spin echo (FSE). Susceptibility artefacts are directly related to field strength.[29] The factors influencing these artefacts are compositions of the material, size and orientation and also the external magnetic field and type of pulse sequence.[30] In order to reduce susceptibility artefacts, GRE sequences should be avoided and, instead, SE or preferably FSE sequences should be used.

Motion Artefacts

These artefacts are caused by discrete movements of the patient. In the cervical spine these artefacts can also be caused by swallowing and in the thoracic spine by cardiac motion.[30] Motion artefacts by swallowing or cardiac movement can be reduced by applying spatial presaturation.

Truncation Artefacts

Truncation artefacts are caused by imperfection in the Fourier transformation. These bright or dark lines are seen parallel to the edges of abrupt intensity changes. These artefacts are more seen on 3-T imaging than in 1.5-T imaging and are a consequence of the improved SNR on 3 T. In the spine these artefacts are especially seen in the interface between spinal cord and CSF, and are a possible cause of overestimation of spinal canal stenosis on MRI. This type of artefact is one of the causes of a band of high or low signal seen near the centre of the spinal cord in mid-sagittal images and is also the source of difficulty for defining the border between the spinal cord and CSF. Their occurrence can be reduced by increasing the spatial resolution (increase matrix size).

Cerebrospinal Fluid Pulsation Artefacts

These artefacts are caused by the pulsatile motion of the cerebrospinal fluid (CSF) caused by to expansion of the CSF during the systolic phase of the cardiac cycle. In the phase-encoding direction this motion can generate linear artefacts parallel to the interface between spinal cord and CSF, producing signal changes in the spinal cord that can be mistaken for intramedullary lesions. Especially in the thoracic spine, areas of turbulent CSF flow related to arachnoidal septa can simulate intradural masses.[31]

REFERENCES

1. Denis F. The three column spine and its significance in the classification of acute thoracolumbar spinal injuries. Spine 1993;8(8): 817–31.
2. Alyas F, Saifuddin A, Connell D. MR imaging evaluation of the bone marrow and marrow infiltrative disorders of the lumbar spine. Magn Reson Imaging Clin North Am 2007;15(2):199–219, vi.
3. Vande Berg BC, Lecouvet FE, Galant C, et al. Normal variants and frequent marrow alterations that simulate bone marrow lesions at MR imaging. Radiol Clin North Am 2005;43(4):761–70, ix.
4. Ricci C, Cova M, Kang YS, et al. Normal age-related patterns of cellular and fatty bone marrow distribution in the axial skeleton: MR imaging study. Radiology 1990;177(1):83–8.
5. Grenier N, Kressel HY, Schiebler ML, et al. Normal and degenerative posterior spinal structures: MR imaging. Radiology 1987; 165(2):517–25.
6. Schellinger D, Wener L, Ragsdale BD, Patronas NJ. Facet joint disorders and their role in the production of back pain and sciatica. Radiographics 1987;7(5):923–44.
7. Xu GL, Haughton VM, Carrera GF. Lumbar facet joint capsule: appearance at MR imaging and CT. Radiology 1990;177(2): 415–20.
8. Schiebler ML, Camerino VJ, Fallon MD, et al. In vivo and ex vivo magnetic resonance imaging evaluation of early disc degeneration with histopathologic correlation. Spine 1991;16(6):635–40.
9. Mahallati H, Wallace CJ, Hunter KM, et al. MR imaging of a hemorrhagic and granulomatous cyst of the ligamentum flavum with pathologic correlation. Am J Neuroradiol 1999;20(6): 1166–8.
10. Xiong L, Zeng QY, Jinkins JR. CT and MRI characteristics of ossification of the ligamenta flava in the thoracic spine. Eur Radiol 2001;11(9):1798–802.
11. Parkin IG, Harrison GR. The topographical anatomy of the lumbar epidural space. J Anat 1985;141:211–17.
12. Tubbs RS, Hallock JD, Radcliff V, et al. Ligaments of the craniocervical junction. J Neurosurg Spine 2011;14(6):697–709.
13. Hanson JA, Blackmore CC, Mann FA, Wilson AJ. Cervical spine injury: a clinical decision rule to identify high-risk patients for helical CT screening. Am J Roentgenol 2000;174(3):713–17.
14. Davis PC, Wippold FJ 2nd, Brunberg JA, et al. ACR Appropriateness Criteria on low back pain. J Am Coll Radiol 2009;6(6): 401–7.
15. Mathen R, Inaba K, Munera F, et al. Prospective evaluation of multislice computed tomography versus plain radiographic cervical spine clearance in trauma patients. J Trauma 2007;62(6): 1427–31.
16. Eberhardt KE, Hollenbach HP, Tomandl B, Huk WJ. Three-dimensional MR myelography of the lumbar spine: comparative case study to X-ray myelography. Eur Radiol 1997;7(5):737–42.
17. Harreld JH, McMenamy JM, Toomay SM, Chason DP. Myelography: a primer. Curr Prob Diagn Radiol 2011;40(4):149–57.
18. Si-jia G, Meng-wei Z, Xi-ping L, et al. The clinical application studies of CT spinal angiography with 64-detector row spiral CT in diagnosing spinal vascular malformations. Eur J Radiol 2009; 71(1):22–8.
19. Nijenhuis RJ, Mull M, Wilmink JT, et al. MR angiography of the great anterior radiculomedullary artery (Adamkiewicz artery) validated by digital subtraction angiography. Am J Neuroradiol 2006;27(7):1565–72.
20. Reith W, Simgen A, Yilmaz U. [Spinal angiography: Anatomy, technique and indications]. Der Radiologe 2012;52(5):430–6.
21. Khanna AJ, Wasserman BA, Sponseller PD. Magnetic resonance imaging of the pediatric spine. J Am Acad Orthop Surg 2003;11(4): 248–59.
22. Dillman JR, Ellis JH, Cohan RH, et al. Frequency and severity of acute allergic-like reactions to gadolinium-containing i.v. contrast media in children and adults. Am J Roentgenol 2007;189(6): 1533–8.
23. Van Goethem JW, Van de Kelft E, Biltjes IG, et al. MRI after successful lumbar discectomy. Neuroradiology 1996;38(Suppl 1): S90–96.
24. Salgado R, Van Goethem JW, van den Hauwe L, Parizel PM. Imaging of the postoperative spine. Semin Roentgenol 2006;41(4): 312–26.
25. Shah LM, Hanrahan CJ. MRI of spinal bone marrow: part I, techniques and normal age-related appearances. Am J Roentgenol 2011;197(6):1298–308.
26. Philpott C, Brotchie P. Comparison of MRI sequences for evaluation of multiple sclerosis of the cervical spinal cord at 3 T. Eur J Radiol 2011;80(3):780–5.

27. Hayes LL, Jones RA, Palasis S, et al. Drop metastases to the pediatric spine revealed with diffusion-weighted MR imaging. Pediatr Radiol 2012;42(8):1009–13.

28. Lavdas E, Vlychou M, Arikidis N, et al. Comparison of T1-weighted fast spin-echo and T1-weighted fluid-attenuated inversion recovery images of the lumbar spine at 3.0 Tesla. Acta Radiol 2010; 51(3):290–5.

29. Parizel PM, van Hasselt BA, van den Hauwe L, et al. Understanding chemical shift induced boundary artefacts as a function of field strength: influence of imaging parameters (bandwidth, field-of-view, and matrix size). Eur J Radiol 1994;18(3):158–64.

30. Vargas MI, Delavelle J, Kohler R, et al. Brain and spine MRI artifacts at 3 Tesla. J Neuroradiol 2009;36(2):74–81.

31. Taber KH, Herrick RC, Weathers SW, et al. Pitfalls and artifacts encountered in clinical MR imaging of the spine. Radiographics 1998;18(6):1499–521.

CHAPTER 2

DEGENERATIVE DISEASE OF THE SPINE

Paul M. Parizel • Thomas Van Thielen • Luc van den Hauwe •
Johan W. Van Goethem

CHAPTER OUTLINE

INTRODUCTION

The spine is a complex anatomical structure composed of vertebrae, intervertebral discs and ligaments. All of these structures may undergo degenerative and morphological changes with age. The intervertebral discs form the connection between two adjacent intervertebral bodies and have two main functions: allowing movement of the spine and to serve as shock absorbers. Movement at a single level is limited; the combined movement of multiple levels allows a significant range of motion. The cervical and lumbar spine, compared with the thoracic spine, has relative more disc height so the motion in these parts is greater. In the posterior region the facet joints play an important role in the cause of neck and low-back pain. Facet joint syndrome is a range of symptoms that cannot be linked to a single nerve root pattern.

DEGENERATIVE DISC DISEASE

Nomenclature and Classification

Since the first description of a 'ruptured disc' by Mixter and Barr in 1934 with monoradiculopathy,[1] the terminology to grade and report degenerative disease of the spine has been controversial and confusing. Some nomenclature systems are based on description of the observed morphology of the disc contour while others include the pathological, clinical and anatomical features. Cross-sectional imaging is based on other definitions and concepts compared to myelography or discography.[2] In 2001

TABLE 2-1 General Classification of Disc Lesions

- Normal (excluding aging changes)
- Congenital/developmental variant
- Degenerative/traumatic lesion
  - Annular tear
  - Herniation
    - Protrusion/extrusion
    - Intravertebral
  - Degeneration
    - Spondylosis deformans
    - Intervertebral osteochondrosis
- Inflammation/infection
- Neoplasia
- Morphological variant of unknown significance

a new nomenclature was proposed by the Combined Task Forces of the North American Spine Society, the American Society of Spine Radiology and the American Society of Neuroradiology which consists of a classification system for the reporting on imaging studies based on pathology.[3] In this chapter we shall follow the general classification of disc lesions as proposed by the Combined Task Forces. The general classification as proposed by Milette is given in Table 2-1.[4]

Age-related Changes in the Intervertebral Disc

The Combined Task Forces reserved the term 'normal' for young discs that are morphologically normal, without

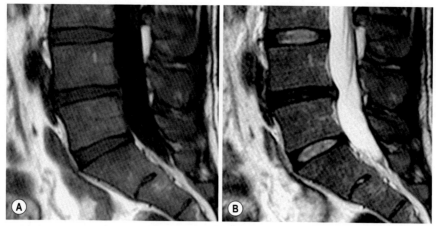

FIGURE 2-1 ■ 'Black disc'. Sagittal T_1 (A) and T_2 images (B) in a 34-year-old man. Decrease in T_2 signal intensity at the level L4–L5 predisposes the disc to degenerative changes.

signs of disease, trauma or ageing. The normal appearance of an intervertebral disc, however, is age-related due to biochemical and anatomical changes which result in a variable appearance on MRI.[5]

In *infants and young children*, the intervertebral disc is prominent relative to the height of the adjacent vertebral bodies. With increasing age the disc volume decreases. The transition between the nucleus pulposus and the annulus is sharp and becomes less distinct with age.[6]

In *young adults* the disc contour coincides with the margins of the adjacent vertebral endplates. On MR imaging the normal adult disc has a low to intermediate signal on T_1-weighted images and a high signal intensity on T_2-weighted images relative to the bone marrow in the adjacent vertebral bodies.[6] On T_2 the bright nucleus pulposus is indistinguishable from the inner annulus. The normal adult endplates, the outer annulus fibrosus and the ligamentous structures are hypointense on T_1 and T_2. The outer annulus is visualised on T_2 and has a low signal intensity.[7] In young adults diurnal changes in T_2 relaxation are present; these changes disappear after the age of 35 years and are thought to be a normal aspect of ageing.[8]

In the *third decade* the intranuclear cleft appears as a horizontal band of decreased signal intensity on T_2 in the central part of the discs, giving it a bilocular appearance on sagittal images. It resembles a fibrous transformation of the gelatinous matrix of the nucleus pulposus.

In *middle-aged and elderly patients* there is a gradual signal loss of the intervertebral discs on the T_2 images until the disc become hypointense.[9] The loss of signal is best seen on T_2 and correlates to a decrease in water and proteoglycan content and increase in collagen. Though the decrease in T_2 signal of the intervertebral disc is age-related it predisposes to degenerative changes in the discs such as loss in disc height, disc herniation and annular tears (Fig. 2-1). The highest T_2 values are seen near the vertebral endplates and the lower T_2 values are present in the intranuclear cleft and the peripheral annulus fibrosus due to its fibrous nature.

In general in the normal ageing disc the height is preserved, disc margins remain regular and radial annular tears are not a usual consequence of ageing. On the basis of a series of post-contrast MRI studies of the lumbar spine, degeneration and normal ageing have been shown to be two separate processes.[10]

Resnick and Niwayama conclude there are two different processes of degeneration: a first type, which can be considered normal ageing, involves the annulus fibrosus and adjacent ring apophysis (spondylosis deformans) (Fig. 2-2); the second type, called intervertebral osteochondrosis, affects the nucleus pulposus and the vertebral endplates, corresponding to the pathological ageing process.[11]

Anterior and lateral marginal osteophytes are considered as normal ageing while endplate changes and reactive bone marrow are seen as pathological changes. Large amounts of gas in the central disc space seen on X-ray or CT studies are indicative for pathological intervertebral osteochondrosis while small amounts of gas near the apophyseal enthesis should be considered as spondylosis deformans (Fig. 2-3).

Degenerative Disc Disease

The prevalence of degenerative disc disease is linearly related to age. Intervertebral disc degeneration begins early in life.[12] Many other factors (e.g. biomechanical and quality of collagen) are also implicated. Degeneration includes changes involving the endplates (sclerosis, defects, Modic changes and osteophytes) as well as disc changes (fibrosis, annular tears, desiccation, loss of height and mucinous degeneration of the annulus).

The relation between low-back pain and abnormalities in the lumbar spine is controversial as abnormal findings are often seen in asymptomatic patients on plain radiographs, CT studies and MRI studies.[13] Degenerative changes in the disc are already seen in one-third of healthy persons between 21 and 40 years old. The high prevalence of asymptomatic disc degeneration must be taken into account when MRI is used for assessment of spinal symptoms.

Although the validity of disc height as an indication for degenerative disc changes is questionable, the loss of height of the intervertebral space is the earliest sign of

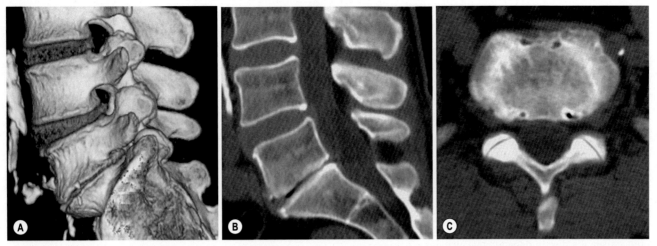

FIGURE 2-2 ■ **Spondylosis deformans ('normal ageing') versus intervertebral osteochondrosis ('abnormal ageing') in a 50-year-old woman.** Three-dimensional (A), sagittal (B) and axial at L5–S1 (C) reformatted CT images. The L5–S1 intervertebral disc is narrowed with irregular endplates, vacuum phenomenon and concentric protrusion of the disc. At the other levels, mild spondylotic changes are seen at the adjacent ring apophysis, indicating normal ageing.

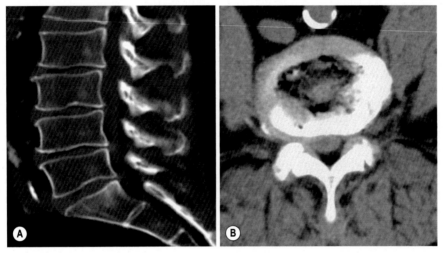

FIGURE 2-3 ■ **Vacuum phenomenon in a 56-year-old man.** Sagittal (A) and axial (B) CT reformatted images. Intradiscal gas at the levels L2–L3 to L5–S1. This so-called vacuum phenomenon is a sign of advanced degeneration.

disc degeneration on plain radiographs. Loss of disc height has been reported in asymptomatic subjects, indicating there is no direct relationship between clinical symptoms and imaging findings. The position of the patient (lying down or standing) should be taken into account.

Other signs, including sclerosis of the vertebral endplates, osteophytes, vacuum phenomenon and calcification, are more reliable, though they indicate late degenerative changes.

Signal loss on T_2 is an early indicator of intervertebral disc degeneration on MRI.[9] As described earlier, in normal ageing the decrease in signal intensity on T_2 should be uniformly distributed over the different levels. If the signal loss is only seen in one or two levels this should be interpreted as abnormal. This finding is often referred to as 'a black disc', and has been applied to describe discogenic pain syndrome (Fig. 2-1). The degenerative process typically starts at the levels with the highest mechanical stress (motion/weight bearing). In the cervical spine, levels C5–C6 and C6–C7 are most commonly involved and in the lumbar spine the levels L5–S1 and L4–L5.

Annular Tears

With ageing, the intervertebral disc becomes more fibrous and less elastic. The degenerative changes are accelerated when the structural integrity of the posterior annulus fibrosus is damaged by overload. This will eventually lead to formation of fissures in the annulus fibrosus. In the international literature the term 'annular tear' is the most widely used and is also supported by the Combined Task Forces; however, the terminology 'annular fissure' is also used. One should take into account that 'annular tear' does not imply this is caused by trauma.

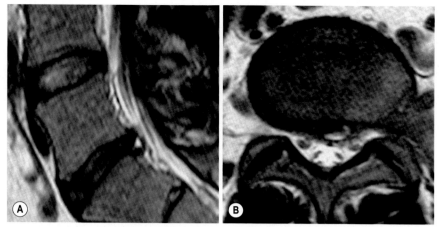

FIGURE 2-4 ■ **Radial annular tear.** Sagittal (A) and axial (B) T_2-weighted images. The radial tear extends to the outer rim of the annulus fibrosus (A). The axial image (B) shows that, in addition, there is a concentric tear involving the outer circumference of the annulus fibrosus. There is a loss of T_2 signal and decrease in disc height at the level L5–S1.

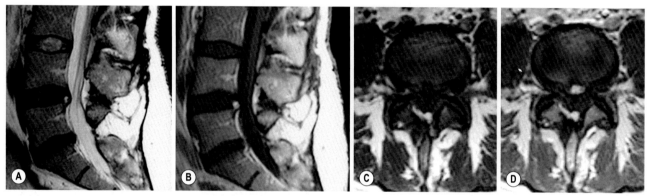

FIGURE 2-5 ■ **Enhancing annular tear.** Pre-contrast sagittal T_2 (A) and axial (C) T_1 images; post-gadolinium sagittal (B) and axial (D) T_1 images. On the T_2 sagittal image a posterior annular tear and central disc herniation is seen at the level L4–L5. After gadolinium administration, there is a linear area of enhancement in the posterior annulus, indicating a concentric tear.

Annular tears can be divided into concentric, transverse or radial tears:[14]

- *Concentric tears* are circumferential lesions found in the outer layers of the annulus fibrosus. Like onion rings, they represent the splitting between adjacent layers of the lamellae annulus. They are believed to be post-traumatic from torsion overload injuries.
- *Transverse tears* or 'rim lesions' are horizontal ruptures of the Sharpey's fibres near the insertion in the bony ring apophysis. The clinical significance of transverse tears remains unclear, although some authors believe they influence and accelerate degeneration and are associated with discogenic pain.[14] They are believed to be post-traumatic in origin and are often associated with small osteophytes.
- *Radial tears* are annular tears permeating from the deep central part of the disc and extend outwards toward the annulus in either the craniocaudal or the transverse plane (Fig. 2-4). Most of these tears do not reach the pain-sensitive outer layers of the annulus. Radial annular tears are associated with disc degeneration[14] and a complete radial tear is necessary for progressive deterioration of the disc.[15]

The clinical significance of annular tears remains unclear. Some annular tears can cause low-back pain without the presence of modification of the disc contours, also known as discogenic pain.[16] On the other hand, annular tears are often found in asymptomatic patients and can be seen as a part of the ageing process.[17]

On MRI annular tears can be seen as an area of high signal intensity on T_2 or as foci of annular enhancement on gadolinium-enhanced T_1[18] (Fig. 2-5). On T_2 the signal intensity is the same as the adjacent cerebrospinal fluid. Repetitive microtrauma may cause annular tears to enlarge and become inflamed; this can be seen as an area of increased signal intensity. This phenomenon is seen on T_2 and is known as a high intensity zone (HIZ).[19] The HIZ is a combination of radial and concentric annular tears which merge in the periphery of the disc. The presence of a high intensity zone is believed to be related to discogenic pain as it involves the outer, highly innervated layers of the annulus. The value of this sign is, however, limited due to a poor sensitivity and a limited positive predictive value.[20] On T_1 extradural inflammation is seen as a zone of intermediate signal intensity, replacing the fat between the disc and the dural sac; on post-contrast images there is intense enhancement.

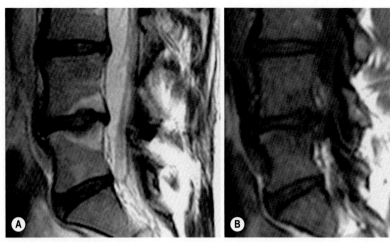

FIGURE 2-6 ■ **Intravertebral herniation at L4–L5.** Sagittal T$_2$ (A) and T$_1$ (B) images. The intravertebral herniations are located in the lower endplate of L4 and the upper endplate of L5. They are surrounded by reactive bone marrow changes, which are hyperintense on the T$_2$ image and hypointense on the T$_1$ image (Modic type I changes).

In the cervical spine annular tears, rim lesions and prolapsed disc material are poorly recognised on MRI, even in severely degenerative disc.[21]

In the thoracic spine herniated disc fragments are often associated with abnormal straight or curvilinear densities on CT, also known as the 'nuclear trail sign'. On MRI this finding may also be associated with a comet-tail configuration in the axial plane. This sign indicates advanced disc disruption and degeneration and must be distinguished from an ageing disc that has not failed.

Disc Heriation

Herniation is defined as a displacement of disc material (cartilage, nucleus, fragmented annular tissue and apophyseal bone) beyond the limits of the intervertebral disc space.[3] The definition of the intervertebral disc is the three-dimensional volume defined by the adjacent vertebral endplates and the outer edges of the vertebral ring apophysis, excluding osteophytes. A break in the vertebral endplates or disruption of the annulus fibrosus is thus necessary for disc displacement to occur. Disc herniations through one or both vertebral endplates are called intervertebral herniations. These herniations are also called Schmorl's nodes and are often surrounded by reactive bone marrow changes (Fig. 2-6). One hypothesis is that this type of herniation is caused by a weak spot in the vertebral endplate caused by regression of the nutrient vascular canals leaving a scar.[22] When in young individuals a herniation of the nucleus pulposus through the ring apophysis occurs before bony fusion a small segment of the vertebral rim may become isolated.[23] This is called a limbus vertebra and is most commonly found in the lumbar region and less frequently on the mid-cervical level. They are characterised by a defect in the anterior wall of the vertebra and usually at the anterior superior margin in the lumbar spine and at the anterior inferior margin at cervical level.

A 'bulging' of the disc is defined as a circumferential or generalised disc displacement involving more than 50% of the disc circumference and is not considered as

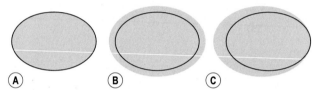

FIGURE 2-7 ■ **Bulging disc.** Symmetrical and asymmetrical bulging disc on transverse CT or MRI images. Normally the intervertebral disc (grey) does not extend beyond the edges of the ring apophyses (black line) (A). In an asymmetrically bulging disc, the disc tissue extends concentrically beyond the edges of the ring apophyses (50–100% of disc circumference) (B). An asymmetrical bulging disc can be associated with scoliosis. Bulging discs are not considered a form of herniation (C).

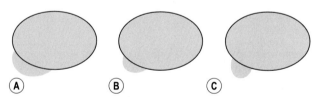

FIGURE 2-8 ■ **Disc herniations.** Types of disc herniations are seen on transverse CT or MRI images. In protrusions: the base of the herniated disc material is broader than the apex. Protrusions can be broad-based (A) or focal (B). In extrusions (C): the base of the herniation is narrower than the apex (toothpaste sign).

being a disc herniation (Fig. 2-7). The term 'bulging' is not correlated with pathology or aetiology but only refers to the morphological characteristics. A bulging can be physiologically seen on the level L5–S1 and on mid-cervical level, can reflect advanced degenerative changes, can be a pseudo-image caused by partial volume effect, can be associated with bone remodelling or can occur in ligamentous laxity.[3] There are two types of disc bulging: an asymmetrical type, as frequently seen in scoliosis, or the symmetrical type, with equal displacement of the disc in all directions.

Two types of disc herniations can be differentiated on the basis of the shape of the displaced disc material (Fig. 2-8). A disc herniation is called an 'extruded disc' when

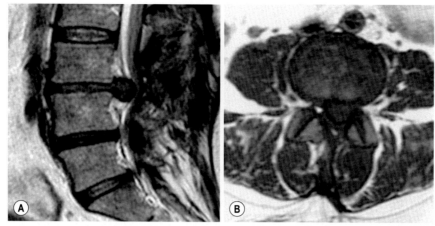

FIGURE 2-9 ■ **Massive disc extrusion.** Sagittal (A) T2 and axial (B) T1 images. A 45-year-old woman with a massive lumbar disc extrusion at L3–L4 with displacement of the nerve roots and obliteration of the left lateral recess. There is also loss of height of the intervertebral disc L3–L4 and decreased signal intensity of the intervertebral disc at L4–L5, indicating degenerative changes.

the base against the disc is smaller than the diameter of the displaced disc material, measured in the same plane (Fig. 2-9). A 'disc protrusion' is used when the base of the disc is broader than any other diameter of the displaced disc material (Fig. 2-10). A protruded disc can be focal if < 25% of the disc circumference is involved or broad-based when 25–50% of the disc circumference is involved.

When there is no connection between the disc and the displaced disc material, this is called a sequestrated fragment or free fragment and is also described as a disc extrusion (Fig. 2-11). On imaging studies, it is often impossible to determine whether continuity exists. Therefore it is more practical to use the term 'migration', which signifies displacement of disc material away from the site of extrusion regardless of the continuity (Fig. 2-12).

The Combined Task Forces have maintained the distinction between protrusion and extrusion, which is useful because an extrusion is seldom seen in asymptomatic patients.[24] The term 'disc extrusion' is also more acceptable to patients than 'disc herniation'.

A 'contained' herniation refers to the displacement of disc material which is covered by the annulus fibrosus. If this cover is absent, the herniation is 'uncontained'. With discography it is possible to distinguish a contained from an uncontained disc herniation and separate a leaking from a non-leaking disc, depending on the displacement of injected contrast agent. On cross-sectional imaging (CT or MRI) it is often impossible to differentiate contained from uncontained disc extrusions.

Communication with clinicians requires an accurate and simple classification of the disc fragments in the vertical and horizontal direction. The Combined Task Forces have opted for a classification based on anatomic boundaries frequently used by surgeons.[25] In the transverse/axial plane the following zones are used:
- central (posterior midline) (Figs. 2-13 and 2-14)
- paracentral (right/left central) (Fig. 2-15)
- right/left subarticular (lateral recess) (Figs. 2-16 and 2-17)

- right/left foraminal (neural foramen) (Fig. 2-10)
- right/left extraforaminal (outside the neural foramen) (Fig. 2-18)
- anterior zone (anterior and anterolateral).

And in the vertical plane from superiorly to inferiorly:
- pedicle level
- infrapedicle level
- disc level
- suprapedicle level.

Spontaneous Regression of Disc Herniation

Spontaneous regression of a lumbar disc herniation is a common finding, although the underlying mechanism remains unclear. Several hypotheses have been proposed: dehydration or shrinkage of the disc, retraction of the disc in the intervertebral space and resorption due to an inflammatory reaction.[26] Free fragment herniation, herniations with peripheral contrast enhancement on T_1 or high signal intensity on T_2 are predisposing for spontaneous regression[27] (Fig. 2-11). Disc material exposed to the epidural space appears to resolve more quickly than subligamentous disc herniations. While contrast enhancement of the posterior longitudinal ligament indicates an inflammatory response, areas of enhancement in the epidural space below or above the herniated disc indicate venous congestion.[28] Strong contrast enhancement indicates an ongoing absorption process and can be used to evaluate disc reabsorption.

Spontaneous regression of a disc herniation has also been described in the cervical spine and only rarely in the thoracic spine. Median or diffuse soft-tissue herniation in the cervical spine is more likely to regress than focal-type herniations.[29]

Vertebral Endplates and Bone Marrow Changes

With ageing, degenerative changes occur in the vertebral endplates and the vertebral bodies; in 1988 Modic

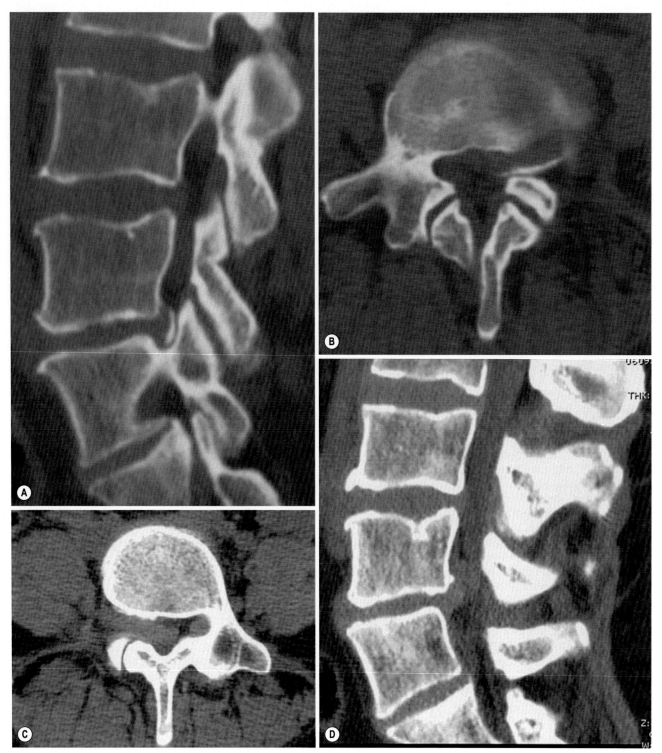

FIGURE 2-10 ■ **Foraminal broad-based disc protrusion.** Sagittal (A) and axial (B) reformatted CT images in bone window setting; sagittal (C) and axial (D) reformatted CT images in soft-tissue window. (A) and (B) show a broad-based foraminal disc protrusion on the left at L4–L5 with a calcified outer rim. At L5–S1 (C, D) there is a broad-based disc protrusion on the right.

described three degrees of degenerative changes in the endplates and the subchondral bone[30,31] (Table 2-2):

- *Type 1 changes* indicate bone marrow oedema with acute or subacute inflammation. This is seen as a decreased signal intensity on T_1 and increased signal on T_2 (Fig. 2-19).

- *Type 2 changes* indicate replacement of the normal bone by fat and are seen as an increased signal on T_1 and iso- to hyperintense on T_2 (Fig. 2-20). Type 2 changes are the most commonly seen.
- *Type 3 changes* are seldom seen and indicate reactive osteosclerosis, seen as a decreased signal on T_1 and T_2.

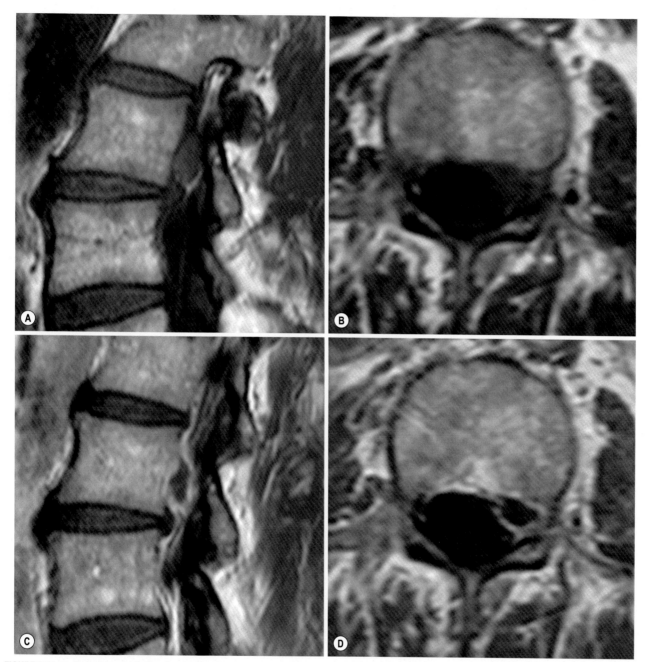

FIGURE 2-11 ■ **Sequestrated disc fragment.** Pre-contrast sagittal (A) and axial (B) T_1 images; post-gadolinium sagittal (C) and axial (D) T_1 images. There is a sequestrated disc fragment posterior to L2. There is a peripheral contrast enhancement on T_1 images post-gadolinium. Peripheral contrast enhancement is associated with a high probability of spontaneous regression.

TABLE 2-2	Signal Intensity Changes in Vertebral Bone Marrow Adjacent to Endplates of Degenerative Discs	
Type 1	↓ SI on T_1 ↑ SI on T_2	Inflammatory stage (bone marrow oedema)
Type 2	↑ SI on T_1 ↑ (or ≈) SI on T_2	Fatty stage (local fatty replacement of bone marrow)
Type 3	↓ SI on T_1 ↓ SI on T_2	Reactive osteosclerosis adjacent to the endplates

SI = signal intensity.

Modic changes are commonly seen on MRI in the bone marrow adjacent to the vertebral endplates. Endplate degeneration may affect one or both endplates. If only a part of the endplates is involved, this is most commonly the anterior part.

Modic type 1 changes indicate an acute inflammatory stage; in most cases these changes transform to type 2 changes over a period of 1–2 years, and can be related to a change in patients' symptoms. This evolution is accelerated after osteosynthesis is performed. Modic type 1 changes are often observed in patients with painful lumbar instability.[32] Type 2 and 3 changes are chronic changes and remain unchanged for years.

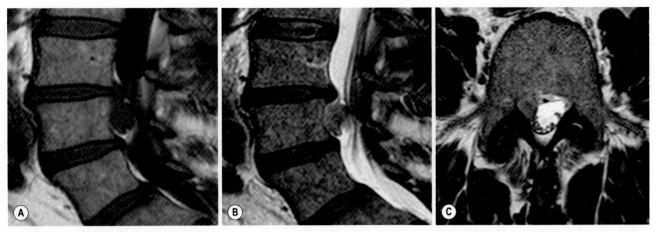

FIGURE 2-12 ■ **Downward migrating disc herniation.** Sagittal T₁ (A), sagittal (B) and axial (C) T₂ images of a 59-year-old man show a large disc fragment descending into the right lateral recess behind the L4 vertebral body. The disc is hypointense on T₂ imaging, indicating a fibrous nature.

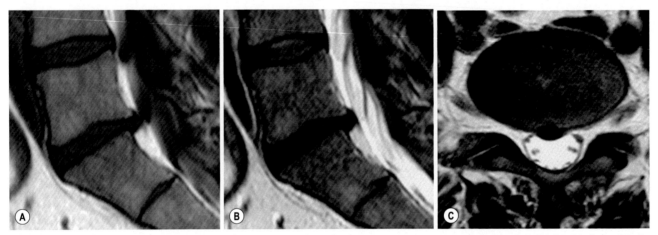

FIGURE 2-13 ■ **Central disc herniation.** Sagittal (A) T₁ image; sagittal (B) and axial (C) T₂ images. Focal central disc herniation at L5–S1 without compression of the nerve roots. The hypointense signal intensity of the disc indicates a fibrous nature.

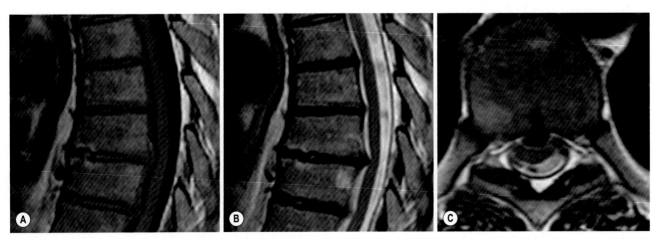

FIGURE 2-14 ■ **Thoracic disc herniation.** Sagittal T₁ (A) image; sagittal (B) and axial (C) T₂ images. Central thoracic disc herniation at the level Th9–Th10. In (C) a small nuclear trail sign is seen.

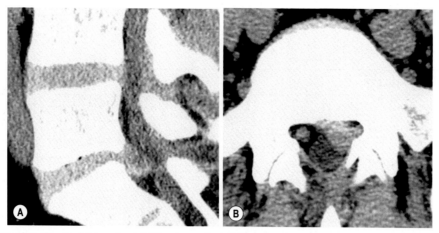

FIGURE 2-15 ■ **Disc extrusion.** Sagittal (A) and axial (B) reformatted CT images show a 42-year-old man with a paracentral disc extrusion on the left side with a descending disc fragment and narrowing of the left lateral recess.

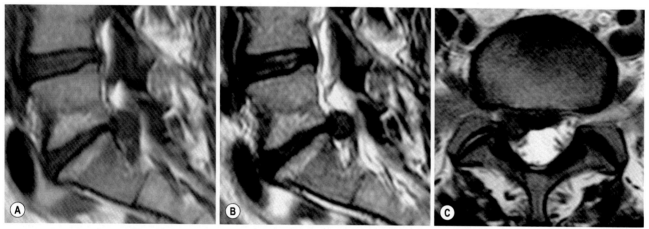

FIGURE 2-16 ■ **Massive lumbar disc extrusion in a 32-year-old woman.** Sagittal T_1 (A) image; sagittal (B) and axial (C) T_2 images. Large subarticular disc extrusion at L5–S1 on the right extending into the right lateral recess. Also note the hyperintense changes in the vertebral endplates at L5–S1 on the T_1 and T_2 images (Modic type 2 changes).

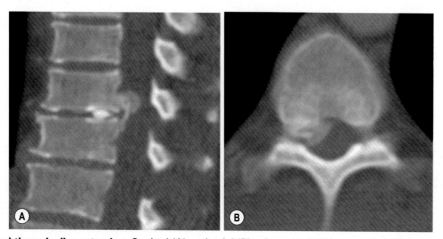

FIGURE 2-17 ■ **Calcified thoracic disc extrusion.** Sagittal (A) and axial (B) reformatted CT images. Calcified ascending disc herniation in the thoracic spine with narrowing of the right lateral recess.

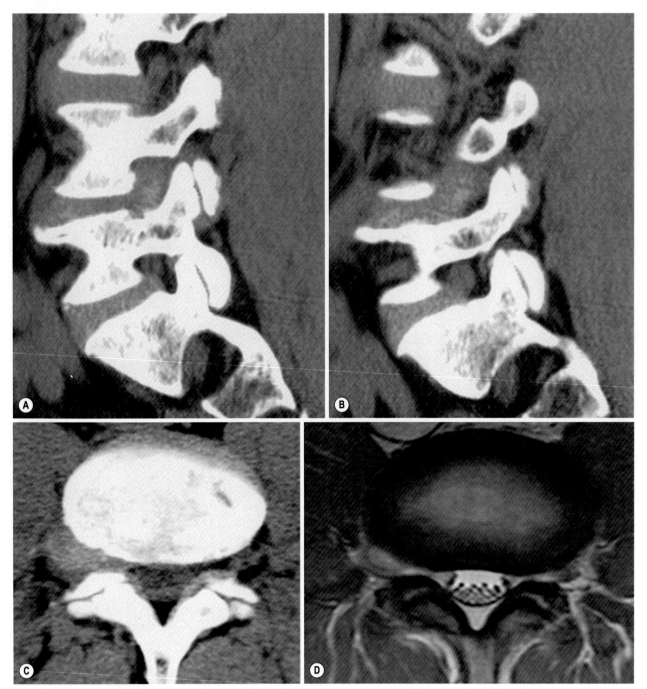

FIGURE 2-18 ■ **Extraforaminal disc herniation.** Sagittal (A, B) and axial (C) reformatted CT images; axial (D) T$_2$ image. A 52-year-old man with an extraforaminal disc herniation on the right side at level L4–L5 extending into the right neuroforamen causing obliteration of the fat in this neuroforamen.

PATHOLOGY OF THE POSTERIOR ELEMENTS

Facet joint syndrome is defined as a range of symptoms that result in diffuse pain that does not follow a clear nerve root pattern. This is described in the cervical as well as in the lumbar spine. In the past the role of the facet joints as a cause of low-back pain has been underestimated. As the synovial linings and joint capsules of

the facet joints are richly innervated, it can be an important source of pain.[33]

As the intervertebral disc and the facet joints work as a three-joint complex, degenerative changes in the disc will change function and anatomy of the posterior elements. On the one hand, facet joint osteoarthritis mostly occurs in the presence of disc degeneration; on the other hand, disc degeneration sometimes occurs without facet joint changes. Therefore, it was suggested that disc degeneration occurs before facet joint

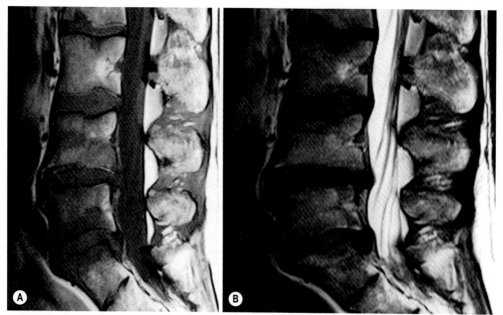

FIGURE 2-19 ■ **Modic type 1 changes.** Sagittal T$_1$ (A) and T$_2$ (B) images. There is a decreased signal intensity on T$_1$ images and increased signal intensity on T$_2$ images in both endplates at level L5–S1 and also in the upper endplate at L4–L5, indicating bone marrow oedema associated with acute or subacute inflammation.

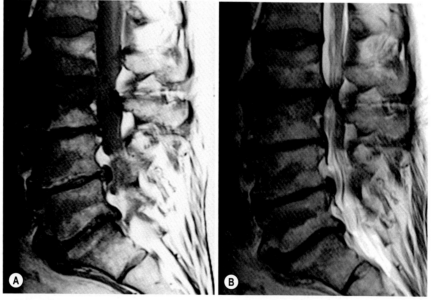

FIGURE 2-20 ■ **Modic type 2 changes.** Sagittal T$_1$ (A) and T$_2$ (B) images. There is an increased signal intensity on T$_1$ and T$_2$ images at L3–L4, L4–L5 and L5–S1, indicating replacement of normal bone marrow by fat. There are also more acute Modic type I changes at L2–L3.

osteoarthritis, possibly secondary to mechanical changes in the loading of the facet joints.[34] Other factors contributing to facet joint degeneration include weight, lordosis and scoliosis.

A significant association was found between sagittal orientation and osteoarthritis of the lumbar facet joints, even in patients without degenerative spondylolisthesis. Boden et al. observed in a study of asymptomatic patients

that more sagittally orientated facet joints at the fourth and fifth lumbar vertebra were associated with herniated discs and spondylolithesis.[35]

Osteoarthritis of the Facet Joints

Degenerative changes of the facet joints are similar to those in peripheral joints and they include osteosclerosis,

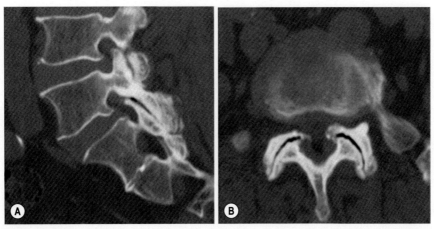

FIGURE 2-21 ■ **Vacuum joint phenomenon in facet joint osteoarthritis.** Sagittal (A) and axial (B) reformatted CT images. Axial CT images show the presence of gas within the L5–S1 facet joints, which may be explained as a result of uneven apposition of the joint surfaces. Associated hypertrophy, juxta-articular calcifications and osteophytes with spinal canal stenosis are present.

thinning of the articular cartilage with erosions and subchondral cyst formation, osteophyte formation, hypertrophy of the articular processes, vacuum joint phenomenon or joint effusion, hypertrophy and/or calcification of the joint capsule and ligamentum flavum.[36] These changes are most commonly found in the lordotic cervical and lumbar segments of the spine.

Hypertrophy is defined as the enlargement of an articular process with normal proportions of its medullary cavity and cortex. This hypertrophy causes distortion of the articular surface, which may cause pain and nerve root compression[36] (Fig. 2-21). Osteophyte formation is an excrescence of bone formation arising from the edges of a joint without a medullary space. Osteophytes protruding ventrally may cause narrowing or stenosis of the lateral canal recesses or the neuroforamina.

Fibrillation and in a later phase fissuring and ulceration of the articular cartilage will develop from the superficial to the deeper layers of the cartilage.[37] In advanced disease the cartilage layers will disappear and subchondral bone sclerosis and cysts will develop. If osteochondral fragments break off the joint surface, these can act as joint mice. Despite the presence of osteophytes and subchondral erosions, the joint space may be preserved. Narrowing of the joint space is frequently observed and may be advanced in patients with facet joint subluxation and erosive osteoarthritis of the facet joint. Widening of the facet joint can be present in severe facet joint degeneration with retrolisthesis due to posterior subluxation.[33]

Weishaupt et al. refined the grading scale of Pathria et al. to grade facet joint osteoarthritis on CT and MRI images[37,38] (Table 2-3, Fig. 2-22).

Standard radiographs including oblique views are a good screening investigation for osteoarthritis of the facet joints although the value is limited.[37,38] The curvature and the double obliquity in the transverse and sagittal plane makes plain film less suited for facet joint imaging as only the portion of the joint parallel to the X-ray beam is visualised. Facet joint narrowing, osteophytes and hyperosthosis may be visualised on standard radiographs as well as spondylolisthesis.

TABLE 2-3   Criteria for Grading Osteoarthritis of the Facet Joints

Grade	Criteria
0	Normal facet joint space (2–4 mm width)
1	Narrowing of the facet joint space (< 2 mm) and/or small osteophytes and/or mild hypertrophy of the articular processes
2	Narrowing of the facet joint space and/or moderate osteophytes and/or moderate hypertrophy of the articular processes and/or mild subarticular bone erosions
3	Narrowing of the facet joint space and/or large osteophytes and/or severe hypertrophy of the articular processes and/or severe subarticular bone erosions and/or subchondral cysts

Both CT and MR imaging have a higher contrast and spatial resolution and are better for evaluating more subtle changes as subchondral erosions and cartilage changes. In general there is a moderate to good agreement between CT and MRI findings. It was, however, demonstrated by Weishaupt et al. that CT is superior to MRI in detecting joint space narrowing and subchondral sclerosis.[37]

Associated Soft-Tissue Changes

Soft-tissue changes associated with facet joint degeneration include degenerative cysts (juxtafacet cysts), ligamentum flavum cysts and hypertrophy and/or calcification of the ligamentum flavum.

Degenerative Cysts Arising from the Facet Joints

Degenerative cysts arising from the facet joints are grouped with the ganglion cysts as juxtafacet or juxta-articular cysts. Ganglion cysts have no connection to the joint and have no synovial lining. These synovial cysts are found periarticular and are attached to the joint by a

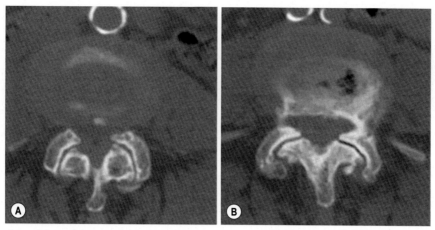

FIGURE 2-22 ■ **Grading facet joint osteoarthritis.** Axial reformatted CT images at L3–L4 (A) and L4–L5 (B). Grade 1 osteoarthritis of the right facet joint L3–L4 (mild hypertrophy) and grade 2 osteoarthritis of the left facet joint (narrowing of the joint space, moderate hypertrophy and osteophytes, subarticular erosion) (A). Grade 3 osteoarthritis of the right facet joint L4–L5 with joint space narrowing, hypertrophy of the articular processes, large osteophytes and subarticular bone erosions can be seen (B).

membrane. The walls are made of loose myxoid connective or fibrocollagenous tissue with a synovial lining and they are filled with yellow or clear mucinous fluid. The consistency of the fluid may vary as haemorrhage and inflammation can be seen.[39]

Juxtafacet cysts are most commonly seen in the lumbar spine and especially at the level L4–L5, which has the most motion in the spine. In the cervical and thoracic spine only a few cases are described. Those in the cervical spine are in half of the cases arising from the cruciate ligament of the atlas.[39] Juxtafacet cysts are increasingly being reported, probably due to the increasing number of MRI examinations performed.[40] Synovial cysts of the facet joints are related to osteoarthritis of the facet joint (Fig. 2-23). The pathogenesis is probably increased motion in the degenerative facet joints. This instability can cause herniation of the synovium through tears in the facet joint capsule.[40] An association between juxtafacet cyst and trauma, chondrocalcinosis, spondylolysis and Baastrup's disease has been reported.

Most juxtafacet cysts arise from the posterior aspect of the facet joint and are situated outside the vertebral canal; anterior cysts into the vertebral canal are four times less frequent.[41]

In the lumbar spine degenerative cysts of the facet joint may cause pain and radicular symptoms by compression of the thecal sac and/or compression of the nerve roots in the lateral recesses. An inflammatory reaction around the juxtafacet cysts may cause sciatica.[40] Depending on the size and location of the cyst, spinal stenosis and/or neurogenic claudication may occur. In the cervical spine facet joint cysts rarely cause radiculopathy.[39]

The natural history of these cysts varies; in a rare case, spontaneous resolution is observed. Haemorrhage is a known complication and causes rapid enlargement, with severe symptoms occurring within months.

In cases of radiculopathy and myelopathy caused by a facet joint cyst, surgery is indicated. Surgical removal is an effective and safe option for treatment. If there is no association with a spinal canal stenosis, a simple excision

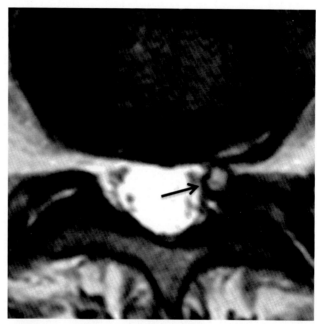

FIGURE 2-23 ■ **Juxtafacet (ganglion) cyst.** Axial T$_2$ image shows a small cystic lesion (arrow) arising from the anteromedial aspect of the left facet joint L5–S1.

of the cyst can be performed. In case of associated spondylotic spinal canal stenosis, a removal of the cyst with decompression and laminectomy may be indicated.[39] An alternative and less invasive technique is the percutaneous injection of local anaesthetics and long-acting steroids.

The typical presentation of a synovial cyst is a rounded mass adjacent to the facet joint with low attenuation. This cyst may show egg-shell calcification of the wall and gas inside.[39]

MRI has a high sensitivity and is the imaging technique of choice.[42] Intraspinal synovial cysts are sharply marginated epidural masses near the facet joint. Typical synovial cysts have a hypointense peripheral rim,

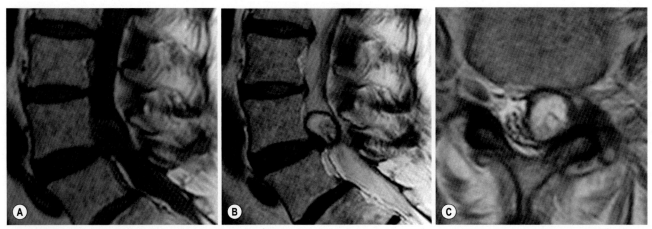

FIGURE 2-24 ■ **Juxtafacet (ganglion) cyst.** Sagittal T_1 (A) image; sagittal (B) and axial (C) T2 images. A large cystic lesion arising from the anteromedial aspect of the left facet joint. The content from the cyst appears mildly hyperintense on T_2 image (B) and is of intermediate signal intensity on T_1 image (A). A low signal intensity rim is observed on the T_2 images (B, C). The cyst causes compression of the thecal sac and obliteration of the left lateral recess is seen.

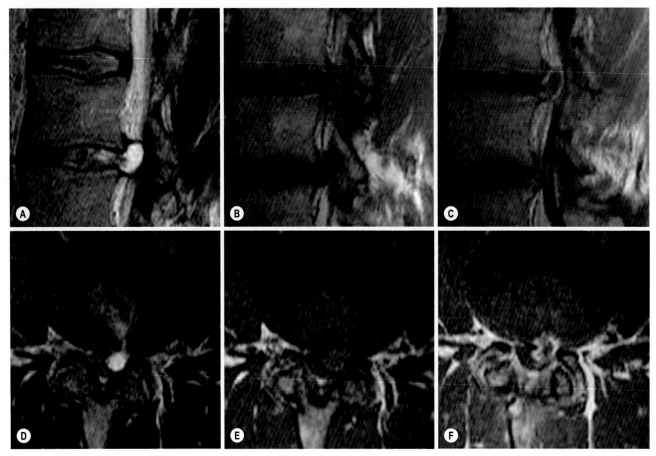

FIGURE 2-25 ■ **Discogenic cyst with narrowing of the left lateral recess.** Sagittal (A) and axial (D) T_2 images; sagittal (B) and axial (E) T_1 images without gadolinium; sagittal (C) and axial (F) T_1 images after gadolinium. Discogenic cyst with hyperintense signal intensity on T_2 images originating from the intervertebral disc L4–L5. This lesion has an intermediate signal intensity on T_1 images and rim enhancement after gadolinium injection. Secondary there is a narrowing of the left lateral recess. Differential diagnosis should be made with a synovial cyst from the facet joints on the basis of its position.

especially on sequences with long TR/TE (Fig. 2-24). This rim enhances after the administration of gadolinium.[43] The signal intensity of a synovial cyst is nearly equal to cerebrospinal fluid on T_1 and on T_2. High signal intensity on T_1 and T_2 indicates subacute blood degradation products.

The differential diagnosis of a mass with this type of signal characteristics in the posterior or lateral spinal canal is broad: juxtafacet cysts, discogenic cysts, cysts of the ligamentum flavum, sequestered disc fragments, infectious cysts or arachnoid cysts and neoplasms (cystic degenerated schwannoma or neurofibroma)[40] (Fig. 2-25).

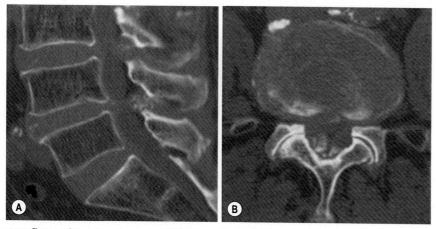

FIGURE 2-26 ■ **Ligamentum flavum hypertrophy and calcification.** Sagittal (A) and axial (B) reformatted CT images. Calcification and hypertrophy of the ligamentum flavum at L4–L5 and in a lesser extend at L3–L4, resulting in a spinal canal stenosis at L4–L5. Calcifications of the ligamentum flavum are also seen in patients with pseudogout. Pseudogout is a crystal-induced arthropathy, which is a debilitating illness in which pain and joint inflammation are caused by the formation of calcium pyrophosphate (CPP) crystals within the joint space. It is sometimes referred to as calcium pyrophosphate disease (CPPD).

Degenerative facet joints are, however, the clue to the most likely diagnosis.

Facet joint arthrography and CT arthrography can be performed if there is any doubt about communication with the adjacent facet joint.

Cysts of the Ligamentum Flavum

Cysts of the ligamentum flavum arise from or are partially embedded in the ligamentum flavum, rather than being close to the facet joints.[40] They are seldom seen and their development may be related to necrosis or myxoid degeneration in a hypertrophied ligamentum flavum.[44] Chronic degenerative changes followed by repeated haemorrhage will form small degenerative cysts; in a later stage these cysts will form one large cyst.[44]

Cyst of the ligamentum flavum are typically located at the level L4–L5, just like juxtafacet cysts. Cysts of the ligamentum flavum have the same imaging characteristics as facet joint cysts. A differentiation may be important, as a simple laminectomy is sufficient for treatment of the ligamentum flavum cysts. On imaging, an extradural, intraspinal mass in close relationship with the ligamentum flavum is seen. On CT imaging, this cyst has a low density compared to the ligamentum flavum. Unlike juxtafacet cysts, no rim calcification has been described.[45] On MR imaging, cysts of the ligamentum flavum are sharply delineated rounded to ovoid cystic masses. They have a high signal intensity on T_2 with a low intensity rim. This rim shows an enhancement after injection of gadolinium.[46]

Ligamentum Flavum Hypertrophy

Symmetrical thickening of the ligamentum flavum is often seen in facet joint arthropathy. It results from facet joint effusion, ligamentous fibrosis, calcification and/or ossification.[47] Degenerative changes are associated with calcifications in the posterior capsule and the ligamentum flavum and the incidence increases with age.[48]

Calcifications of the ligamentum flavum at the insertions are considered normal variants related to traction; calcifications at the periarticular level are thought to be degenerative.[48] Calcifications of the ligament flavum are often seen in patients with diffuse idiopathic skeletal hyperostosis (DISH) and ankylosing spondylitis (Fig. 2-26). They are also observed in patients with metabolic diseases as hypercalcaemia, renal failure, hyperparathyroidism, pseudogout and haemochromatosis.

Calcification of the ligamentum flavum, and especially the posterior longitudinal ligament, is a known cause for radiculopathy and compressive myelopathy in the cervical and thoracic spine (Fig. 2-27). Calcification and/or ossification of the thoracic ligamentum flavum is a rare disease mainly described in the Asian/Japanese literature, and is also known as Japanese disease. Japanese disease mostly affects males younger than 50 years of age. It may cause spinal stenosis with/without myelopathy and/or radiculopathy; the clinical picture consists of progressive myelopathy, resulting in spastic paraparesis.[49] The lower third of the thoracic spine is the most commonly involved, and the cervical spine is only rarely affected. Histopathology of ossification of the ligamentum flavum typically shows mature bone. The ligamentum flavum is progressively replaced by lamellar bone through endochondral ossification. The process starts at the junction between the ligamentum flavum and the joint capsule where a proliferation of cartilaginous tissue triggers ossification.[49]

CT imaging is the imaging technique of choice for evaluating the ossifications. The pathognomonic signs are intense radio-dense lines highlighting the laminae. In most cases these changes are bilaterally present. They usually develop from the medial aspect of the pedicle near the insertion of the ligamentum flavum and progress towards the midline, creating a V-shaped ossification with the anterior concavity situated in the epidural space.[49] Sagittal reconstructions are useful for distinguishing the ossification of the ligamentum flavum from calcifications, which is the only differential diagnosis.

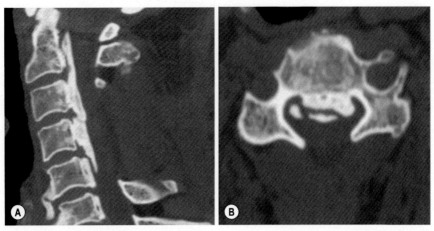

FIGURE 2-27 ■ **Calcification of posterior longitudinal ligament.** Sagittal (A) and axial (B) reformatted CT images show a postoperative condition after posterior laminectomy for a spinal canal stenosis caused by calcifications of the posterior longitudinal ligament from C2 to C5, also known as Japanese disease.

MRI has the advantage of showing changes in the spinal cord as compression of the myelum and myelopathy.

Ossification of the posterior longitudinal ligament is more frequently seen in the cervical spine and less in the thoracic and lumbar spine. Also, thoracic disc herniations may be present in these patients; they also tend to calcify and ossify.[50]

In patients with calcium pyrophosphate dihydrate (CPPD) deposition disease, also known as pseudogout, spinal involvement with calcifications of the ligamentum flavum is rarely seen but may lead to spinal stenosis and spinal cord compression. The lumbar and cervical spine are the most commonly involved. CPPD depositions can also be related to hyperparathyroidism and haemochromatosis.

Degenerative Changes of the Neural Arch

Neural Arch Intervertebral Neoarthrosis

Excessive lumbar lordosis is associated with spine degeneration. Approximation of the adjacent vertebral neural arches may result in abnormal bone contact, resulting in neoarthrosis.[47] Associated remodelling or bony sclerosis of the laminae and pedicles may occur.

Spinous Process Abnormalities and Associated Ligamentous Changes

Baastrup's disease, also known as kissing spine, has been described as a cause of low-back pain (Fig. 2-28). These patients may experience pain caused by irritation of the periosteum or adventitial bursae between abutting spinous processes. It has been described as close approximation and contact of the adjacent spinous processes with enlargement, flattening and reactive sclerosis of the opposing interspinous surfaces.[51] Interspinous bursitis may communicate with the facet joints and can be treated with injection of steroids.

Extension of the synovial cavity to the intraspinal space can result in cyst formation. The cyst can enter the

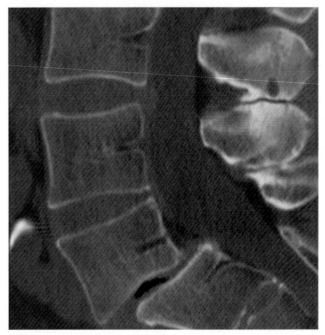

FIGURE 2-28 ■ **Baastrup's phenomenon.** Sagittal reformatted CT image in the midsagittal plane. Grade 2 degenerative spondylolisthesis at the L5–S1 level; malalignment of the spinous processes with anterior slip of the L4 spinous process relative to L5 indicates a type 3 degenerative spondylolisthesis and allows differentiation from isthmic spondylolisthesis. There is collision of the spinous process of adjacent vertebra with progressive interspinous degenerative changes (Baastrup's phenomenon).

epidural space through the midline cleft of the ligamentum flavum to cause extradural compression.[51] Fatty replacement of the paraspinal musculature is often seen in patients with Baastrup's disease.

Degenerative Spondylolisthesis

A spondylolisthesis, also known as an anterolisthesis, is an anterior displacement of a vertebral body relative to the vertebra below. The reverse, when the vertebral body

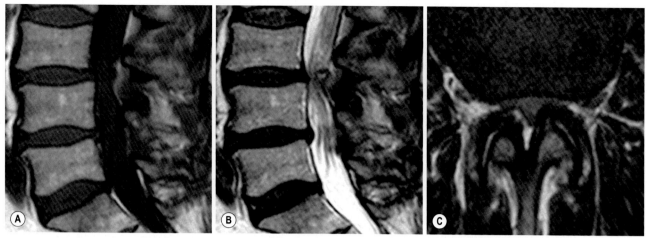

FIGURE 2-29 ■ **Spinal canal stenosis L3–L4 with synovial facet joint cyst.** Sagittal T₁ (A) and sagittal (B) and axial (C) T₂ images. The axial T₂ image shows an hypertrophic facet joint at L3–L4 with a small synovial cyst at the anteromedial aspect of the left facet joint, resulting in a spinal canal stenosis. Also note the discrete anterolisthesis at L3–L4 caused by facet joint osteoarthritis.

below is displaced anteriorly relative to the superior vertebra, is called a retrolisthesis. Six types of spondylolisthesis can be differentiated: congenital dysplasia of the articular processes, defect of the pars articularis, degenerative changes of the facet joint, fracture of the neural arch, weakening of the neural arch due to bone disorders and excessive removal of bone after spinal decompression. Only the degenerative type will be discussed in this chapter.

The most popular grading method is the Meyerding grading system, which divides the anteroposterior diameter of the superior surface of the lower vertebra into quarters, and grades 1 to 4 are assigned to slips of quarters of the superior vertebral body.

Degenerative spondylolisthesis is the most common cause of lumbar spondylolisthesis above the age of 50. This type of spondylolisthesis is caused by degenerative changes of the facet joints. The grade of slippage is usually limited. A more sagittal orientation of the facet joints is typically observed in these patients.[35] As the neural arch is intact, even small progression in the slip may cause cauda equina syndrome. As facet joint osteoarthrosis is most commonly seen at the level L4–L5, spondylolisthesis is also most common at this level. The incidence increases four times if there is a sacralised L5. Women are four times more affected than men.

Clinical symptoms include low-back pain and leg pain as a result of disc and facet joint degeneration, lateral recess and foraminal stenosis leading to nerve root compression. With progression of the spondylolisthesis the symptoms may change from low-back pain to neurogenic claudication due to central canal stenosis.

On imaging, a lateral plain radiograph shows anterolisthesis with degenerative changes at the facet joint and disc space narrowing. Differentiation with isthmic spondylolisthesis can be made by the malalignment of the spinous processes with anterior slip of the spinous process relative to the one of the vertebral body below[52] (Fig. 2-28).

CT and MRI will show osteoarthritis of the facet joints and associated spondylolisthesis. The sagittal orientation of the facet joints, as well as disc degeneration and/or disc bulging, can be evaluated. Sagittal images may demonstrate narrowing of the intervertebral foramina, the lateral recess and/or the central canal with associated compression of the cauda equine and exiting nerve roots. Anterior slip of the inferior articular process will narrow the inferior aspect of the lateral recess and the intervertebral foramen.[52] Associated thickening of the ligamentum flavum may add to the central canal and lateral recess stenosis.

On MRI, bone marrow changes in the pedicle are a non-specific finding of spondylolisthesis and they are often observed in patients with facet joint osteoarthritis. These bone marrow changes are believed to be a response to abnormal stresses related to abnormal motion and loading caused by degenerative changes in the spinal segment.[53]

DEGENERATIVE SPINAL STENOSIS

Degenerative Spinal Canal Stenosis

A stenosis of the spinal canal is a reduction of the diameters of the spinal canal. The normal size of the spinal canal varies according to the location. Spinal canal stenosis may lead to neurological disorders associated with compression of the nervous structures inside the spinal canal (spinal cord, conus medullaris, cauda equina, nerve roots and meninges).

Acquired spinal canal stenosis is the most common type of spinal stenosis at the cervical and lumbar level, and is less frequent in the thoracic spine (Figs. 2-29 and 2-30).

Degenerative changes of the vertebral bodies and facet joints can be associated with degenerative changes of the ligamentous system (calcification and thickening) and herniated discs.

Posterior and central marginal osteophytes can reduce the spinal canal diameter centrally with possible cord compression. In case of multilevel disease the dural sac can get a 'string of pearls'-like appearance on

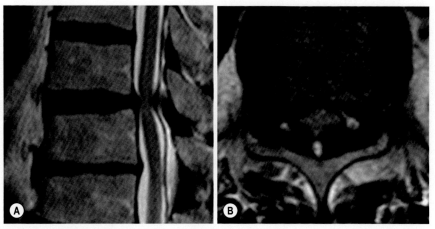

FIGURE 2-30 ■ **Thoracic spinal canal stenosis.** Sagittal (A) and axial (B) T$_2$ images. There is a lateral stenosis of the spinal canal at a low thoracic level due to hypertrophy of the ligamenta flava (B) and a broad-based disc protrusion.

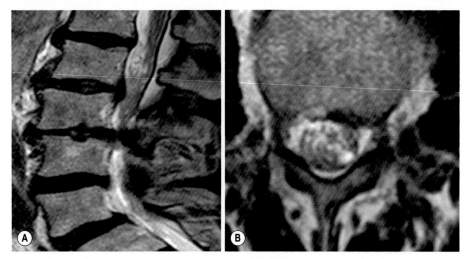

FIGURE 2-31 ■ **Spinal canal stenosis with redundant nerve roots.** Sagittal (A) and axial (B) T2-weighted images. A case of a spinal canal stenosis at L3–L4 as a result of anterolisthesis caused by facet joint osteoarthritis. As seen on the sagittal image (A), it is a case of a concentric spinal canal stenosis with hypertrophy of the ligamenta flava and disc bulging. Proximal of the stenosis there are redundant nerve roots of the cauda equina, as seen on the sagittal (A) and axial images (B).

myelography. A bony protrusion at facet level may cause lateral radicular compression by radicular entrapment in the lateral recess. This phenomenon is more commonly seen at the lumbar level. Disc herniation can also be associated with narrowing of the lateral recess.[54] The compressed nerve root may appear oedematous due to venous congestion and alterations in the blood–nerve barrier.

Posterior and central marginal osteophytosis can lead to the development of a cauda equina syndrome. Compression of the dural sac leads to a reduced space for the nerve roots of the cauda equina. The pressure of the subarachnoidal fluid increases, causing an alteration in the venous drainage, which causes perineural venous congestion and ischaemic damage. Because of its vascular anatomy, the nerve roots of the cauda equina have a higher ischaemic risk if compression is at more than one level. The nerve roots L4, L5 and S1 are predominantly affected. On contrast-enhanced MRI the roots may show enhancement caused by breakdown of the blood–nerve barrier, inflammatory reaction and venous congestion.

With high-grade stenosis in the lumbar spine, the nerve roots proximal to the spinal canal stenosis can be elongated, large and tortuous; this phenomenon is called 'redundant nerve roots' (Figs. 2-31 and 2-32).

Osteoarthritis of the facet joints may cause stenosis of the central spinal canal and the lateral or foraminal recesses. This is most commonly seen at the lumbar level. As described earlier in this chapter, hypertrophy and calcification of the posterior ligaments may also cause stenosis of the spinal canal (Fig. 2-33).

Clinical symptoms of a spinal canal stenosis vary with the level of the spinal stenosis. Patients often remain asymptomatic until an acute event happens. The clinical course of the disease can be influenced by age, sex, socioeconomic situation, site and degree of stenosis.[55] Acute or chronic limb pain and paraesthesias are seen in patients with lateral or foraminal radicular compression. Sensory and motor deficits associated with lower limb pain during walking and in upright position are pathognomonic of lumbar canal stenosis. Forward bending and supine position may relieve the symptoms due to an increase size of

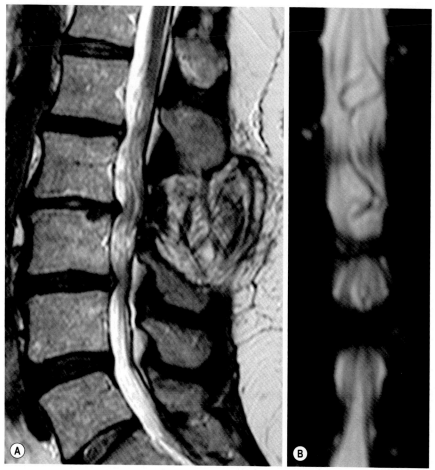

FIGURE 2-32 ■ **Redundant nerve roots.** T$_2$ (A) and MR myelography (B) images. Postoperative status after laminectomy at L2–L3 for a spinal canal stenosis. Sagittal T$_2$ image and the MR myelography shows residual redundant nerve roots of the cauda equina proximal to the previous spinal canal stenosis.

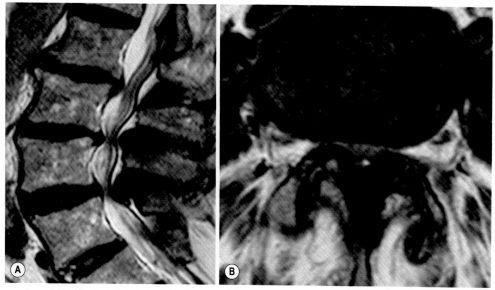

FIGURE 2-33 ■ **Lumbar spinal canal stenosis.** Sagittal (A) and axial at L3–L4 (B) T$_2$ images. Concentric spinal canal stenosis of the lumbar spine at multiple levels (L3–L4 and L4–L5) caused by hypertrophy of the ligamenta flava, concentric disc bulging and hypertrophic facet joint osteoarthritis.

the spinal canal. Vascular claudication and degenerative changes of knee and hip should be included in the differential diagnosis and need to be ruled out. In patients with lumbar spinal stenosis, a neurogenic bladder caused by mechanic compression of the S2–S4 roots can be present due to their location in the posteromedian area of the spinal canal.

Both CT and MRI imaging are non-invasive techniques which make it possible to evaluate the spinal canal. CT is more useful in evaluation of the bony structures. MR examinations used to be limited to the supine position, which cannot always give a clear answer to some clinical conditions. More recently, standing MR equipment has allowed imaging in a weight-bearing environment.

In the past plain radiographs with myelography have been used to evaluate the spinal canal. At this moment this can still be useful to allow dynamic imaging of the spine.

On imaging, the space available for the cord can be determined to evaluate spinal canal stenosis. At the cervical levels C4–C7 the average anteroposterior diameter is 17 mm and values below 14 mm are considered critical. At the cervical level the diameter of the spinal cord is on average 6.9 mm. It can be useful to assess the perimedullar cerebrospinal fluid (CSF) space compared to the sagittal diameter of the spinal cord. If no perimedullar CSF is present, there is a stenosis.

At the lumbar level a classification of spinal stenosis was suggested by Benoist: severe stenosis (< 10 mm), moderate stenosis (10–12 mm) and mild stenosis (12–14 mm).[55] In MRI imaging a severe stenosis is associated with the absence of epidural fat.

Degenerative Foraminal Stenosis

Facet joint osteoarthritis is an important cause of acquired lumbar spinal stenosis. It can cause a stenosis central, lateral and foraminal. In this section we will focus on the foraminal stenosis; degenerative spinal canal stenosis was discussed in the previous section.

The normal intervertebral foramen has a teardrop-like shape, and its form changes significantly in flexion–extension motions as well as in lateral-bending and axial rotation.[56] Foraminal height ranges between 19 and 21 mm and the superior–inferior sagittal diameter ranges between 7 and 8 mm. Instead of measuring the dimensions Wildermuth et al. introduced a qualitative scoring system.[57]

- Grade 0: normal intervertebral foramina; normal dorsolateral border of the intervertebral disc and normal form at the foraminal epidural fat (oval or inverted pear shape).
- Grade 1: slight foraminal stenosis and deformity of the epidural fat, with the remaining fat still completely surrounding the exiting nerve root.
- Grade 2: marked foraminal stenosis, with epidural fat only partially surrounding the nerve root.
- Grade 3: advanced stenosis with obliteration of the epidural fat.

The foraminal width was found to be related to the dimensions of the spinal canal and pedicle length.[58] Disc narrowing significantly reduces the foraminal height but has only little effect on the sagittal dimensions of the intervertebral foramen. Because of the morphology of the lower lumbar vertebrae, the risk of intervertebral nerve root compression is limited in patients with marked disc degeneration and subluxation of the superior facet joint.[58]

Although lateral recess stenosis may be more common than foraminal stenosis, foraminal stenosis with compression of the spinal nerve within the intervertebral foramen is a distinct feature of lateral spinal stenosis.[59] The emerging and exiting nerve root can be compressed at various levels along its descent. Compression of the nerve may be the result of an enlarged superior articular facet or focal osteophytic spurs. Rostrocaudal subluxation of the facet joints will constrict the upper part of the intervertebral foramen and present an obstacle to the nerve root.[33]

Retrolisthesis and isthmic spondylolisthesis may cause foraminal stenosis, while degenerative spondylolisthesis will rather cause lateral or central stenosis by slipping of the inferior articular processes.[58]

Positional pain differences may be related to position-dependent changes in foraminal size and may therefore only be seen in using positional MRI imaging. This technique may show small changes in forms of neural compromise which are not shown in conventional MR imaging.

REFERENCES

1. Mixter WJ, Barr JS. Rupture of the intervertebral disc with involvement of the spinal canal. N Engl J Med 1934;211:210–15.
2. Bogduk N, Modic MT. Lumbar discography. Spine 1996;21(3):402–4.
3. Fardon DF, Milette PC, Combined Task Forces of the North American Spine Society, American Society of Spine Radiology. Nomenclature and classification of lumbar disc pathology. Recommendations of the Combined task Forces of the North American Spine Society, American Society of Spine Radiology, and American Society of Neuroradiology. Spine 2001;26(5):E93–E113.
4. Milette PC. Classification, diagnostic imaging, and imaging characterization of a lumbar herniated disk. Radiol Clin North Am 2000;38(6):1267–92.
5. Sether LA, Yu S, Haughton VM, Fischer ME. Intervertebral disk: normal age-related changes in MR signal intensity. Radiology 1990;177(2):385–8.
6. Yu SW, Haughton VM, Sether LA, Wagner M. Anulus fibrosus in bulging intervertebral disks. Radiology 1988;169(3):761–3.
7. Morgan S, Saifuddin A. MRI of the lumbar intervertebral disc. Clin Radiol 1999;54(11):703–23.
8. Karakida O, Ueda H, Ueda M, Miyasaka T. Diurnal T2 value changes in the lumbar intervertebral discs. Clin Radiol 2003;58(5):389–92.
9. Modic MT, Herfkens RJ. Intervertebral disk: normal age-related changes in MR signal intensity. Radiology 1990;177(2):332–3; discussion 3–4.
10. Rajasekaran S, Babu JN, Arun R, et al. ISSLS prize winner: A study of diffusion in human lumbar discs: a serial magnetic resonance imaging study documenting the influence of the endplate on diffusion in normal and degenerate discs. Spine 2004;29(23):2654–67.
11. Resnick D, Niwayama G. Degenerative disease of the spine. In: Resnick DL, editor. Diagnosis of Bone and Joint Disorders, 3rd ed. Philadelphia: Saunders; 1995.
12. Erkintalo MO, Salminen JJ, Alanen AM, et al. Development of degenerative changes in the lumbar intervertebral disk: results of a prospective MR imaging study in adolescents with and without low-back pain. Radiology 1995;196(2):529–33.

13. Boden SD, Davis DO, Dina TS, et al. Abnormal magnetic-resonance scans of the lumbar spine in asymptomatic subjects. A prospective investigation. J Bone Joint Surg Am 1990;72(3): 403–8.

14. Osti OL, Vernon-Roberts B, Moore R, Fraser RD. Annular tears and disc degeneration in the lumbar spine. A post-mortem study of 135 discs. J Bone Joint Surg Br 1992;74(5):678–82.

15. Herzog RJ. The radiologic assessment for a lumbar disc herniation. Spine 1996;21(24 Suppl):19S–38S.

16. Southern EP, Fye MA, Panjabi MM, et al. Disc degeneration: a human cadaveric study correlating magnetic resonance imaging and quantitative discomanometry. Spine 2000;25(17):2171–5.

17. Boos N, Weissbach S, Rohrbach H, et al. Classification of age-related changes in lumbar intervertebral discs: 2002 Volvo Award in basic science. Spine 2002;27(23):2631–44.

18. Ross JS, Modic MT, Masaryk TJ. Tears of the anulus fibrosus: assessment with Gd-DTPA-enhanced MR imaging. Am J Neuroradiol 1989;10(6):1251–4.

19. Aprill C, Bogduk N. High-intensity zone: a diagnostic sign of painful lumbar disc on magnetic resonance imaging. Br J Radiol 1992;65(773):361–9.

20. Weishaupt D, Zanetti M, Hodler J, et al. Painful lumbar disk derangement: relevance of endplate abnormalities at MR imaging. Radiology 2001;218(2):420–7.

21. Christe A, Laubli R, Guzman R, et al. Degeneration of the cervical disc: histology compared with radiography and magnetic resonance imaging. Neuroradiology 2005;47(10):721–9.

22. Chandraraj S, Briggs CA, Opeskin K. Disc herniations in the young and end-plate vascularity. Clin Anat 1998;11(3):171–6.

23. Mupparapu M, Vuppalapati A, Mozaffari E. Radiographic diagnosis of Limbus vertebra on a lateral cephalometric film: report of a case. Dentmaxillofac Radiol 2002;31(5):328–30.

24. Brant-Zawadzki MN, Jensen MC, Obuchowski N, et al. Interobserver and intraobserver variability in interpretation of lumbar disc abnormalities. A comparison of two nomenclatures. Spine 1995;20(11):1257–63; discussion 1264.

25. Wiltse LL, Berger PE, McCulloch JA. A system for reporting the size and location of lesions in the spine. Spine 1997;22(13): 1534–7.

26. Slavin KV, Raja A, Thornton J, Wagner FC Jr. Spontaneous regression of a large lumbar disc herniation: report of an illustrative case. Surg Neurol 2001;56(5):333–6; discussion 337.

27. Splendiani A, Puglielli E, De Amicis R, et al. Spontaneous resolution of lumbar disk herniation: predictive signs for prognostic evaluation. Neuroradiology 2004;46(11):916–22.

28. Parizel PM, Rodesch G, Baleriaux D, et al. Gd-DTPA-enhanced MR in thoracic disc herniations. Neuroradiology 1989;31(1): 75–9.

29. Matsumoto M, Chiba K, Ishikawa M, et al. Relationships between outcomes of conservative treatment and magnetic resonance imaging findings in patients with mild cervical myelopathy caused by soft disc herniations. Spine 2001;26(14):1592–8.

30. Modic MT, Masaryk TJ, Ross JS, Carter JR. Imaging of degenerative disk disease. Radiology 1988;168(1):177–86.

31. Modic MT, Steinberg PM, Ross JS, et al. Degenerative disk disease: assessment of changes in vertebral body marrow with MR imaging. Radiology 1988;166(1 Pt 1):193–9.

32. Parizel PM, Özsarlak Ö, Van Goethem JWM, et al. The use of magnetic resonance imaging in lumbar instability. In: Szpalski MGR, Gunzburg R, Pope MH, editors. Philadelphia: Lippincott Williams and Wilkins; 1999. pp. 123–38.

33. Schellinger D, Wener L, Ragsdale BD, Patronas NJ. Facet joint disorders and their role in the production of back pain and sciatica. Radiographics 1987;7(5):923–44.

34. Butler D, Trafimow JH, Andersson GB, et al. Discs degenerate before facets. Spine 1990;15(2):111–3.

35. Boden SD, Riew KD, Yamaguchi K, et al. Orientation of the lumbar facet joints: association with degenerative disc disease. J Bone Joint Surg Am 1996;78(3):403–11.

36. Carrera GF, Haughton VM, Syvertsen A, Williams AL. Computed tomography of the lumbar facet joints. Radiology 1980;134(1): 145–8.

37. Weishaupt D, Zanetti M, Boos N, Hodler J. MR imaging and CT in osteoarthritis of the lumbar facet joints. Skeletal Radiol 1999; 28(4):215–19.

38. Pathria M, Sartoris DJ, Resnick D. Osteoarthritis of the facet joints: accuracy of oblique radiographic assessment. Radiology 1987;164(1):227–30.

39. Stoodley MA, Jones NR, Scott G. Cervical and thoracic juxtafacet cysts causing neurologic deficits. Spine 2000;25(8):970–3.

40. Apostolaki E, Davies AM, Evans N, Cassar-Pullicino VN. MR imaging of lumbar facet joint synovial cysts. Eur Radiol 2000; 10(4):615–23.

41. Doyle AJ, Merrilees M. Synovial cysts of the lumbar facet joints in a symptomatic population: prevalence on magnetic resonance imaging. Spine 2004;29(8):874–8.

42. Hagen T, Daschner H, Lensch T. [Juxta-facet cysts: magnetic resonance tomography diagnosis]. Radiologe 2001;41(12):1056–62 [in German].

43. Tillich M, Trummer M, Lindbichler F, Flaschka G. Symptomatic intraspinal synovial cysts of the lumbar spine: correlation of MR and surgical findings. Neuroradiology 2001;43(12):1070–5.

44. Cakir E, Kuzeyli K, Usul H, et al. Ligamentum flavum cyst. J Clin Neurosci 2004;11(1):67–9.

45. Terada H, Yokoyama Y, Kamata N, et al. Cyst of the ligamentum flavum. Neuroradiology 2001;43(1):49–51.

46. Mahallati H, Wallace CJ, Hunter KM, et al. MR imaging of a hemorrhagic and granulomatous cyst of the ligamentum flavum with pathologic correlation. Am J Neuroradiol 1999;20(6):1166–8.

47. Wybier M. Imaging of lumbar degenerative changes involving structures other than disk space. Radiol Clin North Am 2001; 39(1):101–14.

48. Ruiz Santiago F, Alcazar Romero PP, Lopez Machado E, Garcia Espona MA. Calcification of lumbar ligamentum flavum and facet joints capsule. Spine 1997;22(15):1730–4; discussion 1734–5.

49. Pascal-Moussellard H, Cabre P, Smadja D, Catonne Y. Symptomatic ossification of the ligamentum flavum: a clinical series from the French Antilles. Spine 2005;30(14):E400–405.

50. van den Hauwe L, Van Goethem JW, Parizel PM, De Schepper AM. Magnetic resonance imaging of calcified thoracic disk herniation. Eur J Radiol 1993;17(3):148–9.

51. Chen CK, Yeh L, Resnick D, et al. Intraspinal posterior epidural cysts associated with Baastrup's disease: report of 10 patients. Am J Roentgenol 2004;182(1):191–4.

52. Butt S, Saifuddin A. The imaging of lumbar spondylolisthesis. Clin Radiol 2005;60(5):533–46.

53. Morrison JL, Kaplan PA, Dussault RG, Anderson MW. Pedicle marrow signal intensity changes in the lumbar spine: a manifestation of facet degenerative joint disease. Skeletal Radiol 2000;29(12): 703–7.

54. Kanamiya T, Kida H, Seki M, et al. Effect of lumbar disc herniation on clinical symptoms in lateral recess syndrome. Clin Orthop Relat Res 2002;(398):131–5.

55. Benoist M. The natural history of lumbar degenerative spinal stenosis. Joint Bone Spine 2002;69(5):450–7.

56. Fujiwara A, An HS, Lim TH, Haughton VM. Morphologic changes in the lumbar intervertebral foramen due to flexion-extension, lateral bending, and axial rotation: an in vitro anatomic and biomechanical study. Spine 2001;26(8):876–82.

57. Wildermuth S, Zanetti M, Duewell S, et al. Lumbar spine: quantitative and qualitative assessment of positional (upright flexion and extension) MR imaging and myelography. Radiology 1998;207(2): 391–8.

58. Cinotti G, De Santis P, Nofroni I, Postacchini F. Stenosis of lumbar intervertebral foramen: anatomic study on predisposing factors. Spine 2002;27(3):223–9.

59. Fujiwara A, Tamai K, An HS, et al. Orientation and osteoarthritis of the lumbar facet joint. Clin Orthop Relat Res 2001;(385):88–94.

CHAPTER 3

SPINAL TUMOURS

Luc van den Hauwe • Johan W. van Goethem • Danielle Balériaux •
Arthur M. De Schepper[†]

RADIOLOGICAL INVESTIGATIONS IN SPINAL TUMOURS

Computed tomography (CT) and magnetic resonance (MR) imaging are complementary techniques that are needed for evaluation of both the intraosseous extent of the tumour and soft-tissue involvement. MR imaging is the best imaging technique for the evaluation of the epidural space and neural structures.

Plain Film Radiography

Plain film radiography is not the primary imaging technique of choice to image patients with spinal tumours. It is, however, often the first imaging study in the evaluation of patients presenting with back pain. Benign primary bony tumours of the spine are mostly asymptomatic and they are frequently discovered as an incidental finding when plain films are realised on the occasion of a trauma (Fig. 3-1A). Indirect findings that may be associated with intradural spinal tumours are loss of the normal cervical lordosis or torticollis in case of an intramedullary cervical tumour. Scoliosis is almost always present in cases of an extensive spinal cord tumour independent of the histology. These plain film abnormalities are more frequently encountered in children and young adults (58–81%).[1] Indeed, in children, a growing spinal cord tumour (e.g. myxopapillary ependymoma) may expand the bony canal, through pressure erosion, and this enlargement of the spinal canal can be an important feature diagnosed on plain films. Also 'scalloping' of the posterior part of the lower thoracic and upper lumbar vertebrae may be observed in such cases. Intradural extramedullary tumours typically expand into the extradural and paravertebral space. Enlargement of the spinal foramina may be detected on plain films as well as intratumoural calcifications, when present.

Computed Tomography

CT has become the optimal imaging technique for the evaluation of the vertebral bony structures. Multidetector CT (MDCT) allows for rapid and extensive visualisation of the spine and images can be reconstructed in the 3 orthogonal planes. Two-dimensional multiplanar reformatted images are useful in the evaluation of cortical bone destruction and the detection of calcifications (Fig. 3-1B) within the tumour.[2] In case of intradural tumoural pathology, CT may show widening of the bony spinal canal and enlargement of the vertebral neuroforamina. Although CT and MR imaging are diagnostic methods for many cases, CT-guided biopsy may be performed for confirmation, since many bone lesions can have a similar appearance (Fig. 3-2).

Magnetic Resonance Imaging

The imaging technique of choice for the evaluation of spinal tumours is MR imaging (Fig. 3-1C). MR imaging is also very important in the evaluation of lesions of the osseous spine.[3] Protocols may vary slightly between institutions depending on the type of MR system (manufacturer, field strength, etc.), but in general several phased-array coils are used simultaneously to obtain a large field of view.[4] Using advanced parallel acquisition techniques which combine the signals of several coil elements to reconstruct the image, the signal-to-noise ratio is improved along with accelerated acquisition to reduce imaging time. Parallel reconstruction algorithms that reconstruct either the global image from the images produced by each coil, or Fourier plane of the image from the frequency signals of each coil, are used to further improve image quality with better spatial resolution,

---

[†]This chapter is respectfully dedicated to the memory of Professor Dr. Arthur M. De Schepper (1937-2013), who died shortly after the typescript of this chapter was completed.

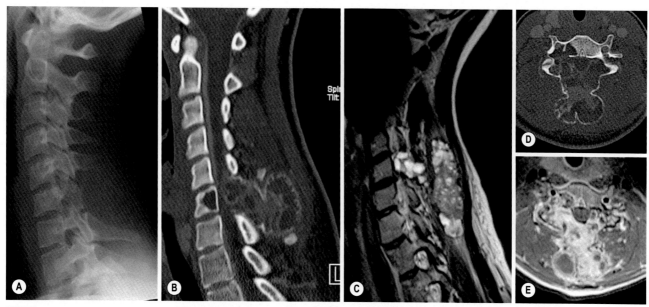

FIGURE 3-1 ■ **Comparison of plain film radiography, MDCT and MR imaging in a patient with a giant cell tumour and secondary aneurysmal bone cyst.** Plain film (A) shows the absence of the C6 spinous process seemingly replaced by a soft-tissue mass, including some slight calcifications and/or remnants of cortical bone. The full extension of the lesion in the spinal canal, the vertebral body, pedicles and posterior elements becomes evident with the use of MDCT (B and D), and MR imaging (C and E). On these T_2-weighted images, fluid–fluid levels can be observed, which are a hallmark for aneurysmal bone cyst (ABC).

FIGURE 3-2 ■ **CT-guided percutaneous biopsy of a vertebral tumour with important paravertebral extension.** Sagittal contrast-enhanced T_1 (A) and axial fat-suppressed T_2 (STIR) (B) show the tumour mass extending within the paravertebral soft tissues and anterior epidural space with a typical 'curtain sign'. CT-guided percutaneous biopsy of the large paravertebral mass is performed with the patient in prone position (C). Pathology demonstrated low-grade chondrosarcoma. (Case courtesy of P. Bracke, Brasschaat, Belgium.)

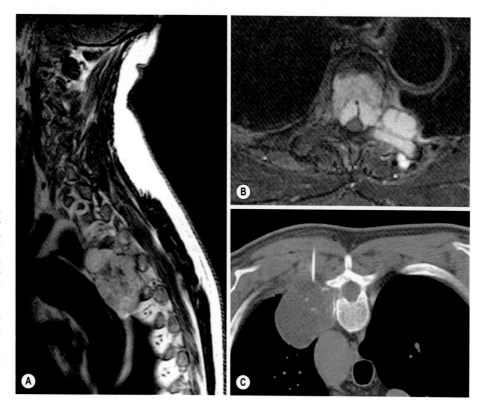

and reduced artefacts.[5] Full-spine and whole-body MR imaging can be performed in this manner. This is important, since it is advantageous to see the whole spine and spinal cord covered in one single examination (Fig. 3-3).

Imaging protocols usually include sagittal and axial T_1 and T_2. T_1 and T_2 offer different and complementary information. T_2 is superior in detecting intramedullary tumours. On the other hand, T_1 is more sensitive than non-fat-suppressed T_2 in detecting bone marrow disease, e.g. vertebral metastases, but short T_1 inversion recovery (STIR) or other fat-suppressed T_2 sequences are also able to increase the detection of certain bone marrow diseases. Suppressing the high signal of CSF in T_2 sequences is

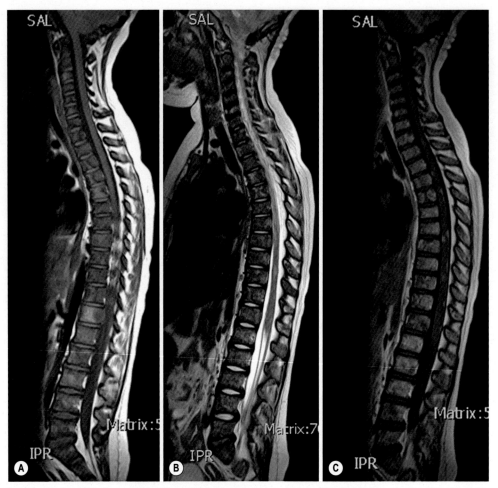

FIGURE 3-3 ■ **Full-spine MR imaging in a child with recurrent and metastatic medulloblastoma.** Sagittal T_1 (A) shows diffuse hetero-geneous signal intensity within the bone marrow of the cervical, thoracic and lumbar vertebrae, indicative of metastatic bone disease. On sagittal T_2 (B), an ill-defined area of high signal intensity within the spinal cord is observed at the Th9–Th10 level with suspicion of more intramedullary lesions more proximally. Sagittal gadolinium-enhanced T_1 (C) not only shows diffuse leptomeningeal enhancement but also confirms the presence of intramedullary metastases and shows enhancement of the vertebral metastases.

very useful in detecting subtle intramedullary lesions. The most common technique to obtain this kind of image is FLAIR (fluid-attenuated inversion recovery), a sequence that nulls out CSF signal. Gradient-echo (GRE) images are useful in order to detect haemorrhagic components often present in spinal cord tumours. In screening for vertebral metastases, an additional sagittal GRE so-called out-of-phase sequence can be used. In the normal adult human, the medullary bone of the vertebral bodies contains approximately equal amounts of water and fat protons. In out-of-phase conditions, the signal of both will cancel out, leaving the vertebrae completely black. In case of vertebral pathology, however, the signal will increase and, as such, vertebral metastases (or other lesions) will clearly stand out.[6] Gadolinium-enhanced sequences, usually performed in the sagittal and axial plane, are used in order to better identify solid enhancing tumour components, and to differentiate tumoural cysts whose borders enhance from associated, so-called reactive, pseudocysts.[7,8] Coronal images may be helpful for the evaluation of paravertebral soft-tissue extension and fat suppression can be used to better demonstrate

tumoural enhancement.[2] Some authors recommend contrast-enhanced 3D-GRE T_1 techniques in screening for intradural tumour dissemination.[9] When dealing with extradural tumours, the administration of gadolinium is also useful for biopsy in that it allows differentiation of enhancing viable tumour from areas of non-enhancing necrosis (Fig. 3-2). Moreover, gadolinium-enhanced images better demonstrate epidural extension of the tumour.[2]

Diffusion-Weighted Imaging

Diffusion-weighted imaging (DWI) and diffusion tensor imaging (DTI) have been proven useful in brain tumours. However, these techniques are much more difficult to apply in imaging of the spinal cord. Obtaining spinal cord DWI and DTI has a number of challenges. The spinal cord's small size requires the use of small voxel sizes (higher matrix) for spatial resolution that decreases the signal-to-noise ratio. Images may be degraded because of macroscopic motion related to physiological cerebro-spinal fluid pulsations, breathing and swallowing. In

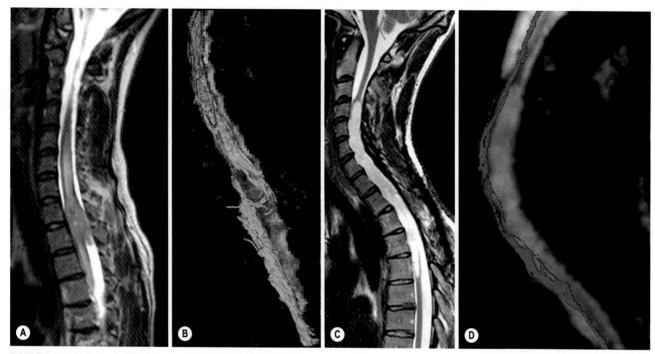

FIGURE 3-4 ■ **Value of diffusion tensor imaging (DTI) tractography.** Sagittal T_2 (A) and DTI tractography (B) in a patient with spinal cord ependymoma. Peripheral displacement rather than tumoural invasion of the fibres is observed. Sagittal T_2 (C) and DTI tractography (D) in a patient with spinal cord astrocytoma. Fibres are pushed anteriorly by the tumour. (Case (A, B) courtesy of M. Thurnher, Vienna, Austria and W. Van Hecke, Leuven, Belgium.)

addition, local field inhomogeneities reducing the image resolution and the use of echo-planar sequences, typically used in brain imaging, further increases susceptibility effects.[10] Although still under development, fibre tracking based on DTI holds great potential in visualising the fibres within the normal and diseased spinal cord. The effect of a growing spinal cord tumour on the fibre tracts has been demonstrated. If the lesion displaces the fibre tracts rather than infiltrating them it is is suggestive of a well-circumscribed tumour such as ependymoma (Fig. 3-4A, B), which pathologically has a plane of resection between the lesion and the normal spinal cord allowing for a surgical resection compared with a diffusely infiltrating tumour such as fibrillary astrocytoma.[10–13]

Bone Scintigraphy

Bone scintigraphy can be performed when multifocal vertebral lesions with increased radionuclide uptake are suspected. However, bone scintigraphy is limited in its capacity to depict detailed surgical anatomy, particularly compared with CT or MR imaging.[2] Moreover, positive findings may also be attributed to degenerative changes of the spine.

Positron Emission Tomography

Positron emission tomography (PET) has been used extensively to evaluate the grade of malignancy in brain tumours and to differentiate recurrent tumours from

radiation necrosis after radiation therapy. In other regions, PET has been used to detect neoplastic lesions such as metastatic ones, and to differentiate neoplastic from non-neoplastic lesions.[14] Only a few reports on the use of PET in patients with intramedullary tumours have been published. Wilmshurst et al. reported the use of both ^{18}F-fluorodeoxyglucose (FDG) and ^{11}C-methionine (MET) and found a correlation with histological malignancy.[15] FDG-PET imaging is also useful in evaluating tumour progression and identifying the most metabolically active components in spinal cord tumours. A prospective study of larger numbers of patients with a wider range of tumour types is required, but this is difficult to achieve given the rarity of spinal cord tumours.[14,15]

CLASSIFICATION OF SPINAL TUMOURS

Spinal tumours may be classified in different ways. The World Health Organisation (WHO) classification of spinal tumours is a universally accepted histological classification. The 2007 WHO classification is based on the consensus of an international Working Group of 25 pathologists and geneticists, as well as contributions from more than 70 international experts overall, and is presented as the standard for the definition of CNS tumours to the clinical oncology and cancer research communities worldwide.[16] The WHO classification of CNS neoplasms is based on the assumption that the tumour type results from the abnormal growth of a specific cell type. The WHO classification also provides a grading system for tumours of each cell type and allows the classification of tumours to guide the choice of therapy and predict prognosis. Based on the grading system, most tumours are of a single defined grade. Although the updated WHO classification does not have a direct impact on the daily practice of the (neuro)radiologist or in the interpretation of images, it is valuable in the communication between clinicians, radiologists and pathologists.[4,16]

Based on their location on imaging findings (MR imaging, and myelography in the past), spinal tumours may be characterised as intramedullary, intradural extramedullary, and extradural spinal tumours.[17] Although this classification is somewhat of an oversimplification, since lesions can reside in several compartments, this approach is very helpful as it narrows the differential diagnosis when a tumour is found in one of these anatomical compartments. Extradural lesions are the most common (60% of all spinal tumours), with the majority of lesions originating from the vertebrae. Metastatic disease is the most frequent extradural tumour, while primary bone tumours are much less frequently observed. Intradural tumours are rare, and the majority are extramedullary (30% of all spinal tumours), with meningiomas, nerve sheath tumours (schwannomas and neurofibromas) and drop metastases being the most frequent ones. Intramedullary tumours are even more uncommon lesions (10% of all spinal tumours). Astrocytomas and ependymomas comprise the majority of the intramedullary tumours.[6]

Intramedullary Tumours

Primary tumours of the spinal cord are 10 to 15 times less common than primary intracranial tumours and overall represent 2 to 4% of all primary tumours of the central nervous system (CNS).[17] They occur with an incidence of 1.1 cases per 100,000 persons. A considerable number of different intramedullary tumours exist; only a few of them are expected to be encountered in a routine practice. The majority of intramedullary tumours are glial tumours; about 90% are ependymomas or astrocytomas. The most frequently encountered neoplasms in adults are ependymoma (40–60%) and astrocytoma. Haemangioblastoma is the third most frequent intramedullary tumour found in adults, but it is rarely seen in children. Astrocytomas are the most common intramedullary tumour in the paediatric age group (60–90% of cases), followed by gangliogliomas. Ependymomas are uncommon in children outside the setting of neurofibromatosis type 2 (NF-2).[18] Astrocytomas and ependymomas are more frequent in the thoracic and the cervical region, respectively, while myxopapillary ependymomas are typically seen in the region of the conus medullaris, filum terminale and cauda equina.[5,6]

MR imaging is the preoperative study of choice to narrow the differential diagnosis and guide surgical resection.[19] Differentiation between ependymomas and astrocytomas before surgery is important for the surgeon because ependymomas of the spinal cord are relatively well circumscribed and they can apparently be completely removed, whereas astrocytomas have a tendency for infiltrating growth that makes complete removal difficult.[20]

Ependymoma

Ependymomas are the most frequent intramedullary tumours in adults; in children these tumours occur sporadically and may be associated with NF-2. Most NF-2-related ependymomas are small intramedullary nodules that may be multiple.[18] The peak incidence for spinal ependymomas is in the fourth and fifth decade, but these tumours also are found in younger patients. Ependymomas arise from the ependymal cells lining the central ependymal canal and, therefore, are frequently located centrally within the cord.[7] This central location explains the more frequently observed sensory symptoms that result from the close proximity to the spinothalamic tracts.[21] Motor deficits only present in the later stage of the disease, thereby delaying the diagnosis. In contrast to sporadic tumours, the majority of NF-2-related spinal tumours are asymptomatic.[22] Intramedullary ependymomas are most often found in the cervical cord and less frequently also the upper thoracic cord. Most ependymomas are low grade (WHO grade 2) with a benign indolent course. The tumours are well demarcated and compress the adjacent cord rather than infiltrating it. Malignant histological subtypes (anaplastic ependymoma; WHO grade 3) rarely occur. There are four histological subtypes of CNS ependymomas: cellular, papillary, clear cell and tanycytic.[6] The cellular form is the most common intramedullary variant.[21] The prognosis for patients with spinal ependymoma depends on the tumour grade, degree of resection and presence or absence of CSF dissemination.[21] In NF-2-patients, these tumours seldom require intervention, even for tumours that expand the cord or have associated cysts. Close surveillance with MR imaging is a reasonable option.[22]

CT may show canal widening, scoliosis and vertebral body scalloping. On MR imaging, ependymomas appear typically as central well-circumscribed iso- or hypointense lesions on T_1 (Fig. 3-5A) and as iso- or hyperintense on T_2 (Fig. 3-5B).[21] Most ependymomas do enhance vividly (Fig. 3-5C) and homogeneously in 91% of the cases. They have usually well-defined borders (Figs. 3-5C, 3-6A), which allows total removal of the tumour in most cases (Fig. 3-6B).[8] Because of their compressive rather than infiltrative nature, a cleavage plane may occasionally be seen on imaging. Diffusion tensor imaging may show how the tumours displace the fibre tracts rather than interrupt them (Figs. 3-4A, B). However, this may also be observed in spinal cord astrocytoma (Figs. 3-4C, D). While astrocytomas usually are very extensive, the mean tumour size of ependymomas is usually three vertebral segments. A so-called 'cap sign' is seen in 20–25% of cases and corresponds to low signal intensity areas seen on T_2 and even better on gradient-echo T_2^*, capping at both sides the tumour limits (Fig. 3-6A). Those caps are haemosiderin deposits due to chronic haemorrhage. When present, the cap sign is highly suggestive for the diagnosis of ependymoma.[21] Associated satellite cysts are seen in 60% of the cases, and they may be very large. Delineation of these cysts is easier after gadolinium injection. Syrinx is also a characteristic finding, especially with cervical ependymomas. Spinal cord oedema on either side of the tumour

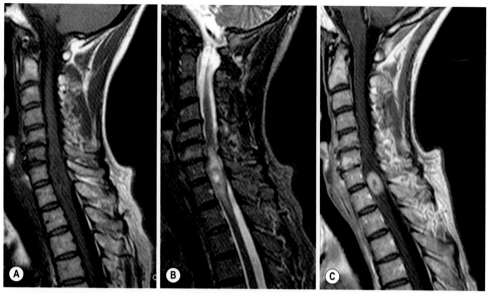

FIGURE 3-5 ■ **Spinal cord ependymoma.** Sagittal T_1 (A) and T_2 (B) show clearly focal spinal cord enlargement at the cervicothoracic junction. The lesion is iso- to slightly hypointense on T_1, and very heterogeneous on T_2 with areas of low signal intensity within the tumour. There is some associated oedema within the cord. Gd-enhanced T_1 (C) shows focal nodular contrast enhancement centrally within the spinal cord. Straightening of the spine and multilevel degenerative changes of the lower C-spine are observed.

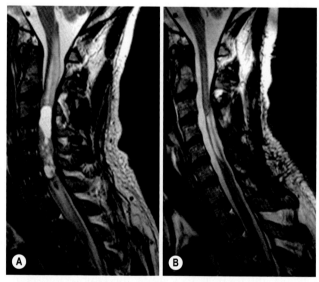

FIGURE 3-6 ■ **'Cap sign' in a grade 2 ependymoma.** Preoperative sagittal T_2 (A) shows an expansile lesion arising within the spinal cord at the C3–C7 level. Heterogeneous signal intensity of the tumour with both solid and cystic components. The most typical feature is the bilateral hypointense areas capping the tumour: the 'cap sign' is more frequently encountered in ependymoma. Extensive oedema is observed. Postoperative sagittal T_2 (B) shows complete removal of the tumour.

is variable, but often seen in the large multisegmental tumours.[4]

Myxopapillary Ependymoma

Myxopapillary ependymoma, a WHO grade 1 lesion, is a relatively common spinal intradural neoplasm of the conus medullaris and filum terminale arising from ependymal cells of the filum terminale. It is found

predominantly in children and young adults, although it may be observed at older age. There is a slight male preponderance. Patients typical complain of chronic low back pain exacerbating during night. Myxopapillary ependymomas are slow-growing tumours, so they may become very large before the diagnosis is finally made. Associated scalloping of the vertebral body, scoliosis and enlargement of the neural foramina may be observed. Haemorrhage may occur, explaining the sudden worsening of clinical symptoms with occurrence of leg weakness and sphincter disturbances. This greater tendency for haemorrhage may also lead to subarachnoid bleeding and superficial siderosis.

On MR imaging, the lesion is iso- to hyperintense on T_1 (Fig. 3-7A) and hyperintense on T_2 (Fig. 3-7B). The hyperintense signal may be explained by their mucin content. The tumour enhances strongly and is somewhat inhomogeneous after gadolinium injection (Fig. 3-7C). Haemorrhage and cyst formations are common features that contribute to signal inhomogeneity.

The main differential diagnosis is with nerve sheath tumours, such as schwannomas.[18] Although myxopapillary ependymomas are WHO grade 1 lesions, spontaneous and postoperative CSF dissemination along the craniospinal axis as well as dissemination following extradural manipulation of the tumour during spine surgery or following spinal trauma has been reported.[23] In our experience, postoperative radiotherapy is therefore very useful to prevent recurrent disease.

Astrocytoma

Astrocytomas are the most common intramedullary tumours (up to 90%) in children[18] and account for about 30% of intramedullary tumours in adults. The peak incidence for spinal astrocytomas is in the third and fourth decade.[4,6] A slight predominance among males (55%) is

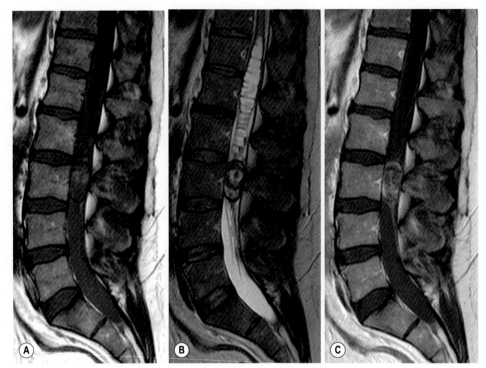

FIGURE 3-7 ■ **Myxopapillary ependymoma.** Sagittal T_1 (A) and T_2 (B) show a well-defined heterogeneous mass at the L3 level. The lesion is slightly hyperintense on T_1, which may be explained by the presence of mucin, but it shows low signal on T_2, and has a low signal intensity rim, suggestive for haemorrhage within the tumour. Inferior to the mass, trapped CSF has high T_1 and T_2 signal, possibly caused by a high protein content. Extensive cyst formation with enlargement of the spinal cord is observed proximal to the tumour with some oedema at the border with the normal cord. Sagittal gadolinium-enhanced T_1 (C) shows enhancement of the tumour mass.

observed in larger series. Histology is the most important prognostic variable. In the paediatric age group, astrocytomas are mostly tumours of low grade (i.e. pilocytic and fibrillary astrocytomas).[19] Pilocytic astrocytomas (WHO grade 1) account for 75% of all intramedullary tumours in the paediatric age group and typically affect children between 1 and 5 years of age, whereas fibrillary astrocytomas (WHO grade 2) account for 7% and tend to occur in older children (around 10 years of age).[18] In adults, the majority (75%) are low-grade (WHO grade 2) fibrillary astrocytomas with 5-year survivorship exceeding 75%. High-grade spinal cord gliomas (WHO grades 3 and 4) are less common and associated with a poor survival. Regardless of WHO grade, spinal cord astrocytomas are infiltrative and associated with poorly characterised boundaries and, consequently, are typically biopsied only since total resection is not possible.[17] The most common site of involvement is the thoracic cord (almost 70%), followed by the cervical cord. They frequently involve a large portion of the spinal cord, spanning multiple vertebral levels in length (Fig. 3-8). Involvement of the entire spinal cord (holocord presentation) is common in children but quite rare in adults.[24] True 'holocord' tumours, however, are rare. In most cases, involvement of the whole length of the spinal cord is caused by extensive spinal cord oedema rather than by a tumour.

Tumours can show areas of necrotic-cystic degeneration (60% of cases), can have a 'cyst with mural nodule' appearance, or can be structurally solid (about 40% of cases). The solid components are iso- to hypointense on T_1 (Fig. 3-9A) and hyperintense on T_2 (Fig. 3-9B), whereas necrotic-cystic components are typically hypointense on T_1 and strongly hyperintense on T_2. The pattern of enhancement is variable and does not define tumour margins.[18] For the most part, low-grade fibrillary astrocytomas do not enhance (Fig. 3-9C), although enhancement may be observed (Fig. 3-8C). Low-grade tumours may evolve over time and become more malignant tumours. Pilocytic astrocytomas, on the other hand, do enhance intensely as they do in the brain. High-grade astrocytomas and glioblastomas tend to be more heterogeneous with necrotic-cystic areas and enhance often in a patchy mode. Intratumoural haemorrhage may be observed and is best seen on gradient-echo T_2^*. Associated syringomyelia may occur: the borders of those associated cavities do not enhance after contrast injection (Fig. 3-8C).

Haemangioblastoma

Haemangioblastomas are rare benign (low grade), usually richly vascularised tumours. They represent 2–10% of all spinal tumours and are seen more commonly in adults, with a peak incidence in the fourth decade.[25] Hemangioblastomas can be solitary (80%) or multiple (20%), when associated with von Hippel–Lindau syndrome (VHLs).[26,27] This is an autosomal dominant disease with multiple cerebellar and/or spinal haemangioblastomas (Fig. 3-10),

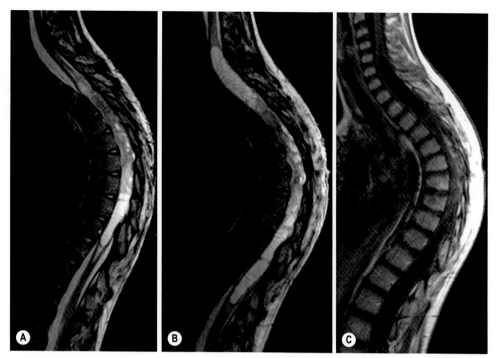

FIGURE 3-8 ■ **Spinal cord astrocytoma.** Follow-up study with sagittal T$_2$ (A, B) in an 11-year-old girl who had partial resection of the tumour 2 and 3 years before, respectively. Final diagnosis at that time was grade 2 fibrillary astrocytoma. Progressive enlargement of the associated polar cysts proximal and distal to the resected tumour is observed. Also the spinal cord oedema has increased. Sagittal contrast-enhanced T$_1$ of the most recent follow-up study (C) shows heterogeneous enhancement, not present on the previous examination, which is indicative of progressive disease. Note the hyperkyphosis and scoliosis in this girl, which are frequently indirect signs of intradural spinal tumours in children.

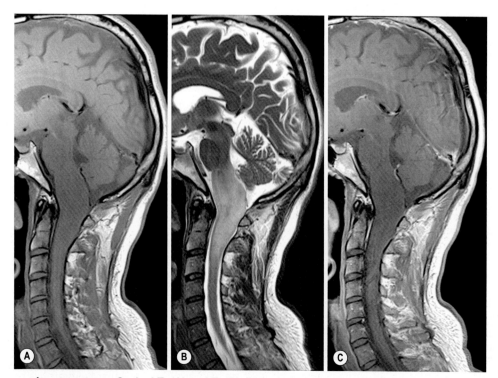

FIGURE 3-9 ■ **Low-grade astrocytoma.** Sagittal T$_1$ (A) and T$_2$ (B) show an ill-defined mass with huge swelling of the upper cervical spinal cord and medulla oblongata just extending up to the level of the bulbomedullary junction and even higher in the posterior aspect of the brainstem. Signal characteristics are aspecific, with diffuse low signal intensity on T$_1$ and high signal intensity on T$_2$. Sagittal contrast-enhanced T$_1$ (C) shows no enhancement within the lesion.

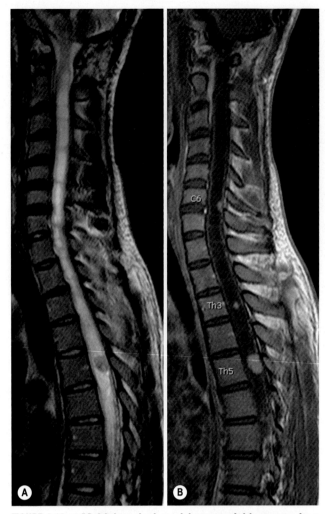

FIGURE 3-10 ■ **Multiple spinal cord haemangioblastomas in a patient with von Hippel–Lindau syndrome.** Sagittal T₂ (A) shows a diffuse enlarged spinal cord with a slight hypointense nodular lesion at the posterior aspect (subpial) of the spinal cord at the Th5 level. The lesion is surrounded by extensive oedema and multiple associated cysts can be observed proximal to the tumour. Sagittal gadolinium-enhanced T₁ (B) shows strong enhancement within the tumour. Moreover, two smaller additional enhancing nodules at the level of the C6–C7 disc space and Th3 are found. Associated peritumoural cysts show no enhancement.

retinal angiomatosis, renal cell carcinoma and/or phaeochromocytoma in varying degrees.[27] Spinal hemangioblastomas associated with VHLs are usually diagnosed up to 10 years earlier and are associated with less severe neurological symptoms than sporadic lesions. The incidence of spinal haemangioblastomas may be as high as 88% in patients with VHLs,[28] which is much more frequent than previously reported.[29] Therefore, screening spinal MR imaging should be performed in patients with VHLs. Most patients with sporadic disease have a single lesion at the cervical or thoracic level (Fig. 3-11), whereas patients with VHLs have multiple lesions at all spinal levels (Fig. 3-10). Up to one-third of patients with VHLs will develop new lesions every 2 years.[28]

In about 75–85% of cases these are pure intramedullary lesions, but sometimes they may be intradural extramedullary with a variable exophytic component. Pure extradural tumours are very rare.[30] Preoperative evaluation of the precise tumour location is important for total resection and improving the surgical outcome.[30] Haemangioblastomas have two different but rather typical presentations: either a small nodular lesion located in the subpial region and surrounded by extensive intramedullary oedema or a small nodule associated with huge and extensive intramedullary cystic components (Figs. 3-10 and 3-11). The mechanism of this peritumoural cyst formation appears to be the result of an interstitial process that starts with generation of oedema. Vascular endothelial growth factor (VEGF) acting locally in the tumour or hydrodynamic forces, or both, within abnormal tumour vasculature may drive fluid (plasma) extravasation. When these forces overcome the ability of the surrounding tissue to resorb fluid, oedema (with its associated increased interstitial pressure) and subsequent cyst formation occur.[31]

On T₁, the solid tumour nodule is isointense to hypointense relative to the spinal cord; on T₂ it is isointense to slightly hyperintense. A rich vascular network in the tumour, as well as enlarged feeding arteries and dilated draining veins (Figs. 3-11B–D), may best be seen on proton density and T₂. After gadolinium injection, intense and homogeneous enhancement of the subpial nodule is seen.[8] Gadolinium is especially useful in order to pick up small, multiple nodules when associated with large cystic components (Fig. 3-10B). Associated cysts may have signal intensities comparable to CSF, but sometimes a rich protein content results in a higher signal intensity on T₁. Symptomatic small haemangioblastomas have relatively large associated syringes, whereas asymptomatic ones do not.[32] DSA is still performed to identify the feeding arteries to the tumour (Figs. 3-11E, F) and, if possible, to perform preoperative embolisation in order to reduce the bleeding during surgery of those richly vascularised tumours.

Ganglioglioma

Gangliogliomas, being rare tumours in adults (1–2% of all spinal cord tumours),[33] are much more frequently seen in children.[21,34] They represent the second most common intramedullary tumour in the paediatric age group (15% of cases) and mostly affect children between 1 and 5 years of age, as do pilocytic astrocytomas.[18] These tumours are composed of a combination of neoplastic ganglion cells and glial elements. Although they typically are low-grade tumours (WHO grades 1 and 2) with a low potential for malignant degeneration, they have a significant propensity for local recurrence, and the glial element may progress to high grade.[18] Surgical resection is the treatment of choice. After resection, there is a 5-year survival rate of 89%. Their preferential location is in the cervical and upper thoracic cord and may extend to the medulla oblongata through the foramen magnum.[18] Gangliogliomas may extend over more than eight vertebral segments[19] and holocord involvement has been described to be more frequent than in other spinal cord tumours, probably as a result of their slow growth rate.[34] Gangliogliomas are typically eccentrically located (Fig. 3-12).[21]

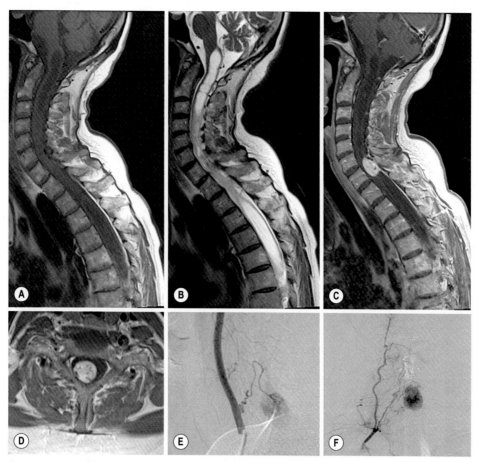

FIGURE 3-11 ■ **Cervical haemangioblastoma.** Sagittal T_1 (A) and T_2 (B) show a diffuse enlargement of the spinal cord. Extensive oedema and multiple cyst formation can be seen extending up to the level of the obex. Sagittal (C) and axial (D) gadolinium-enhanced T_1 show the presence of an intense enhancing tumour at the C7 level. Flow voids can be observed within the enhancing tumour. Enhancement is also visible in dilated veins along the posterior aspect of the spinal cord. DSA (E, F) shows the typical hypervascularisation supplied by enlarged arterial branches arising from the right vertebral and right thyrocervical trunk. (Case courtesy of M. Voormolen, Antwerp, Belgium.)

On imaging, scoliosis and remodelling are common but non-specific findings.[18] Calcification may be seen on CT, but it is much less common than in gangliogliomas that occur intracranially. According to Rossi et al., calcification is probably the single most suggestive feature of gangliogliomas. In the absence of gross calcification, the MR imaging appearance of gangliogliomas is non-specific and does not allow differentiation from astrocytomas.[18] Gangliogliomas have highly variable MR imaging findings. Although propensity for cyst formation has been reported to be common,[19] in other series gangliogliomas were predominantly solid.[18] In a large series of 27 patients with spinal cord gangliogliomas, Patel et al. described several clinical and imaging findings that are characteristic of gangliogliomas: young patient age, long tumour length, tumoural cysts (Fig. 3-12B), absence of oedema, mixed signal intensity on T_1, patchy tumour enhancement (Fig. 3-12C) and cord surface enhancement.[33] They speculated that the mixed signal intensity on T_1 may be caused by the dual cellular population (i.e. neuronal and glial elements) and, in their opinion, this feature was somewhat unique for spinal neoplasms and was uncommonly seen in cord ependymomas or

astrocytomas.[33] Perifocal oedema can vary from limited or absent to extensive. Contrast enhancement can be focal or patchy, and it rarely involves the whole tumour mass;[18] absence of enhancement has also been described in a minority of cases.[35]

Less Frequent Intramedullary Tumours

Less frequent tumours include intramedullary metastasis, lymphoma, epidermoid cyst, lipoma, oligodendroglioma, intramedullary schwannoma and teratoma.

Metastasis. Although intramedullary metastases are rare, accounting for only 5% of all intramedullary lesions, their number is growing fast due to the longer survival of many cancer patients (improved chemotherapy, etc.). They are less common than leptomeningeal metastases. The lung and breast are the most common sites of primary malignancies for intramedullary spread.[4] The high sensitivity of MR imaging enables easy detection of intramedullary metastases: however, there are no specific MRI characteristics. Usually, spinal cord metastases are small, nodular, well-defined lesions, surrounded

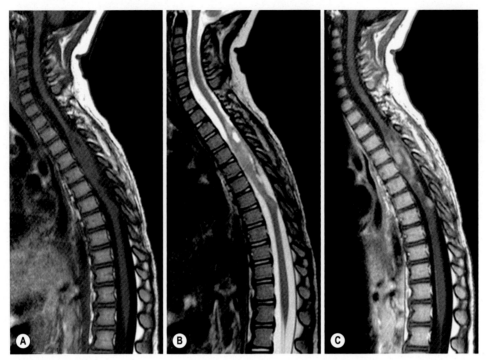

FIGURE 3-12 ■ **Ganglioglioma.** Sagittal T_1 (A) and T_2 (B) show a heterogeneous solid infiltrating tumour in a young child, arising within the thoracic spinal cord, and extending along 5–6 segments. Small intratumoural cysts and discrete peritumoural oedema may be observed on the T_2. Diffuse heterogeneous and patchy enhancement of the tumour is present on sagittal T_1 after gadolinium injection (C). (Case courtesy of A. Rossi, Genoa, Italy.)

by mild to extensive oedema (Fig. 3-13A). The enhancement pattern may be either ring-like or homogeneous and intense (Fig. 3-13B).[36] Recently, two peripheral enhancement features on MR imaging specific for non-CNS-origin spinal cord metastases have been described: a more intense thin rim of peripheral enhancement around an enhancing lesion (rim sign) and an ill-defined flame-shaped region of enhancement at the superior/inferior margins (flame sign).[37] Melanoma metastasis has a more specific appearance, exhibiting a spontaneously hyperintense aspect on T_1 linked to the presence of melanin.

Spinal Cord Tumour Mimics

It may be difficult or impossible to differentiate spinal cord tumours from intramedullary non-neoplastic lesions. In one series of 212 patients undergoing surgery for intramedullary spinal cord 'tumours', Lee et al. reported 4% of non-neoplastic lesions.[38] A variety of lesions may mimic a spinal cord tumour such as vascular cavernous malformations (cavernomas) (Fig. 3-14), tumefactive demyelinating lesions in multiple sclerosis (MS), neuromyelitis optica (NMO) (Fig. 3-15) and acute disseminating encephalomyelitis (ADEM), acute transverse myelitis (ATM), spinal cord contusion and spinal cord infarction. Also, sarcoidosis and vasculitis may mimic a spinal cord tumour. The clinical picture, laboratory findings, electrophysiological testing, and, finally, additional MR imaging of the brain may help to recognise these entities properly, in order to avoid unnecessary biopsy.

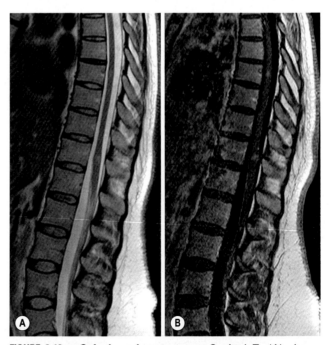

FIGURE 3-13 ■ **Spinal cord metastases.** Sagittal T_2 (A) shows two discrete areas of high signal intensity centrally within the spinal cord at the Th8 and Th11 levels. There is no obvious spinal cord oedema. Sagittal gadolinium-enhanced T_1 (B) shows enhancement of the lesions in this 35-year-old woman with advanced breast carcinoma. MR imaging of the brain, performed at the same time (not shown), demonstrated multiple brain metastases in both cerebral and cerebellar hemispheres.

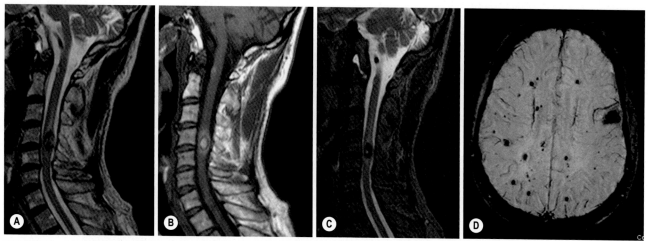

FIGURE 3-14 ■ **Multiple cavernomas in a patient with familial cavernomatosis.** Sagittal T_2 (A), sagittal T_1 (B) and sagittal GRE T_2* (C). The typical 'mulberry' or 'popcorn' aspect, typical white and black aspect of this C4–C5 lesion. A small, at the C2 level. cavernous malformation, especially on the T_2. This imaging sequence best demonstrates the signs of chronic bleeding within the lesion. There is no perilesional oedema. The lesion is spontaneously partly hyperintense on T_1 and enhances moderately after contrast administration. Axial susceptibility-weighted imaging (SWI) of the brain (D) shows numerous cavernomas.

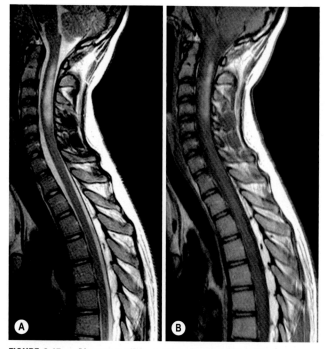

FIGURE 3-15 ■ **Neuromyelitis optica.** Sagittal T_2 (A) shows an ill-defined area of high signal intensity extending across 3–4 spinal segments; mild enlargement of the spinal cord is noticed. Sagittal gadolinium-enhanced T_1 (B) shows patchy enhancement of the lesion. Knowledge of a clinical history of neuritis optica and normal MR imaging findings of the brain enable the correct diagnosis to be made.

Cavernous Malformation (Cavernoma). Cavernous malformations (also known as cavernous angiomas, or cavernomas) represent 7–10% of all intramedullary tumours. They most commonly involve the thoracic spinal cord segments. These vascular malformations may remain clinically silent for a long period of time before an acute and rapidly progressive neurological deficit

occurs due to bleeding. Before the advent of MR imaging, these lesions were extremely difficult to diagnose, especially in the spinal cord, as they usually are small and do not enlarge the spinal cord. Intramedullary cavernous malformations are usually easily recognised thanks to the typical 'black and white' or 'popcorn' appearance due to areas of mixed signal intensity on both T_1 and T_2 or T_2* (Figs. 3-14A–C). Contrast enhancement is variable. As patients with spinal cord cavernomas tend to have multiple other malformations elsewhere in the neuraxis, and also a higher association with familial cavernomatosis, we recommend performing MR imaging of the brain (Fig. 3-14D) whenever the diagnosis of an intramedullary cavernous malformation is suspected.[39]

Intradural Extramedullary Tumours

Intradural extramedullary tumours result in displacement of the cord to the contralateral side and widening of the ipsilateral CSF space. Patients with intradural extramedullary neoplasms frequently present with progressive myelopathy. Weakness is the most common symptom, and diffuse back pain or radicular pain may be present. Most intradural extramedullary tumours are benign. They originate either in a spinal nerve or from the meninges. The differential diagnosis for lesions in this location is limited and can be further narrowed with knowledge of specific imaging characteristics.[40]

Meningiomas and nerve sheath tumours make up for about 90% of all extramedullary intradural tumours. Schwannomas are the most common intradural extramedullary tumours. In the paediatric population, the most common intradural extramedullary neoplasms are leptomeningeal metastases resulting from primary brain tumours.[18,40] Primary tumours in this location are less frequently observed and are mostly schwannomas and neurofibromas in NF-2 and NF-1 patients, respectively.[18]

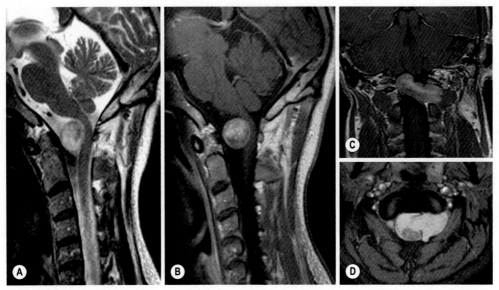

FIGURE 3-16 ■ **Upper cervical neurinoma in a patient with neurofibromatosis type 1.** Sagittal (A) and axial (D) T_2 show a well-delineated mass with high signal intensity. The spinal cord is displaced posteriorly and is compressed by the tumour, which extends through the left C2–C3 neuroforamen. Sagittal (B) and coronal (C) gadolinium-enhanced T_1 show intense contrast enhancement. The axial and coronal planes best show the typical dumbbell aspect of spinal neurinomas involving both the intra- and extradural space, and facilitate discrimination between neurinoma and meningioma (see Fig. 3-20).

Nerve Sheath Tumours: Schwannoma and Neurofibroma

Schwannomas, aka neurinomas or neurilemmomas, are considered benign tumours (WHO grade 1) and represent the most common intradural extramedullary tumours. Schwannomas are usually solitary (Fig. 3-16) and are more commonly seen in adults. Although far less common in children, multiple schwannomas occur in children with NF-2[41] (Fig. 3-17). In these patients the risk of malignant transformation is higher. Typically, schwannomas arise from the dorsal sensory nerve roots.[42] The vast majority (70%) of schwannomas are purely intradural extramedullary tumours, 15% are extradural and 15% have a 'dumbbell' shape involving both the intra- and extradural space (Fig. 3-16). Schwannomas are mostly found at the cervical and lumbar region and less frequently at the thoracic level. On MR imaging, schwannomas are usually well-encapsulated tumours that may have cystic components. They are usually iso-intense to the spinal cord in most cases while some 20% are moderately hypointense on T_1. On T_2, schwannomas are hyperintense (Fig. 3-16A). Calcification and haemorrhage are rare. Contrast enhancement may vary and can be intense and homogeneous or only show faint peripheral enhancement (Figs. 3-16–3-18).[42] Giant schwannomas are typically encountered at the lumbar level and it may be difficult sometimes to discriminate them from myxopapillary ependymoma.[43,44] The distribution of the roots of the cauda equina in the thecal sac on axial imaging may help in distinguishing these tumours: a myxopapillary ependymoma of the filum pushes the roots to the periphery of the thecal sac, whereas a schwannoma of the cauda more often pushes the roots together in an eccentric fashion.[44]

Neurofibromas are not well encapsulated, are ill-defined and often present as multiple tumours. MR imaging usually does not enable differentiation between schwannoma and neurofibroma when the tumour is solitary. In NF-1, multiple plexiform neurofibromas are typically encountered: they are iso-/hyperintense on T_2 and a 'target sign' (hyperintense rim with low/intermediate centre) may be observed. Enhancement is usually mild. Malignant degeneration may occur rarely, mainly in the case of NF-2.

Meningioma

Meningiomas are mainly dural-based intradural tumours. More than 95% of meningiomas are benign tumours (WHO grade 1). They are the second most common intraspinal tumours, occurring most frequently in older patients (peak age in the fifth and sixth decades).[4] Meningiomas are uncommon tumours in the paediatric age group outside the setting of NF-2.[18,40] Overall, 80% of meningiomas are found in the thoracic region, with a female preponderance. In men, however, only half of the meningiomas are in the thoracic region and another 40% are cervical. Meningiomas are mostly located posterolaterally in the thoracic region (Fig. 3-19) and anteriorly in the cervical region (Fig. 3-20).[6] They are usually solitary tumours, but multiple meningiomas, which occur in 2% of affected patients, are most often associated with NF-2.[41] Meningiomas are very slowly growing and major cord compression may be seen with only minor symptoms.

On CT, meningiomas are iso- to hyperattenuating. The hyperattenuation reflects the cellular nature of these lesions, but the presence of calcification also contributes. Hyperostosis may be seen but is not as common as in the

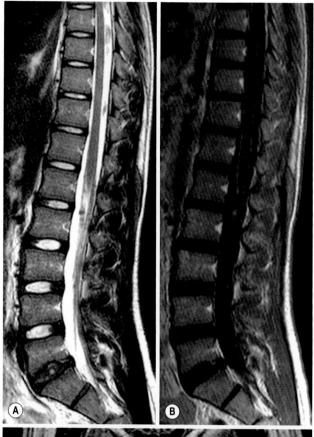

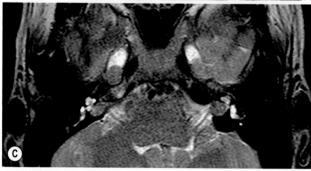

FIGURE 3-17 ■ **Multiple schwannomas in a young boy.** The MR examination was performed to further characterise a subcutaneous lesion at the L1 level, which was observed clinically. Sagittal T_2 (A) shows some discrete, small nodules attached to the nerve roots of the cauda equina. On sagittal (B) gadolinium-enhanced T_1, many more of these lesions can be observed and show intense contrast enhancement. Axial brain T_2 (C) at the level of the internal auditory canals shows bilateral vestibular nerve schwannomas, pathognomonic for the diagnosis of neurofibromatosis type 2. Bilateral trigeminal nerve schwannomas located within Meckel's cave can be observed.

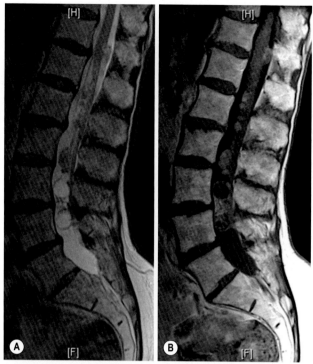

FIGURE 3-18 ■ **Multiple neurofibromas in a young woman with neurofibromatosis type 1.** Sagittal T_2 (A) and sagittal gadolinium-enhanced T_1 (B) show multiple bulky and nodular tumours arising from spinal nerve roots which are a typically representation of neurofibromatosis type 1. They are iso- to hyperintense on T_2 and show strong homogeneous enhancement. MR imaging of the complete neuraxis is mandatory in the work-up of neurofibromatosis patients.

intracranial forms. This is due, in part, to the more prominent epidural fat within the spine.[40] On MR imaging, meningiomas are iso- to hypointense on T_1 and slightly hyperintense on T_2. There is a strong and homogeneous enhancement with gadolinium (Figs. 3-19B, C and 3-20C, D), except for the calcified areas. Some meningiomas are heavily calcified and dark on all sequences with only little contrast uptake. The classical 'dural tail' may be seen (Figs. 3-19B and 3-20C, D) although this aspect is less frequently and less typically found in the spine compared to the intracranial location.[42] Meningiomas may cause compression and displacement of the spinal cord (Figs. 3-19 and 3-20). Signal changes in the spinal cord secondary to compression can be seen (Fig. 3-21C), but are usually rare.[4]

Metastases

Leptomeningeal metastases are secondary tumours that may arise from a malignant primary neoplasm outside the CNS, such as a breast, lung or other neoplasm (Fig. 3-21), or from the spread of a CNS tumour, i.e. the so-called 'drop metastasis'. Common primary CNS tumours that may spread to the leptomeninges are medulloblastoma (Fig. 3-3), choroid plexus papilloma and carcinoma, ependymoma and high-grade glioma. Leptomeningeal dissemination from CNS neoplasms occurs in younger patients, whereas metastases from lung or breast carcinomas are more frequently observed in older patients.[4] MR imaging is more sensitive than CSF cytology for the detection of subarachnoid spread of primary brain tumours, though CSF cytology may be more sensitive for CSF spread of leukaemias and lymphomas.[45,46] Contrast-enhanced series are the imaging technique of choice to assess for metastasis. Leptomeningeal metastases demonstrate three patterns of enhancement: (1) diffuse contrast enhancement along the pia of the

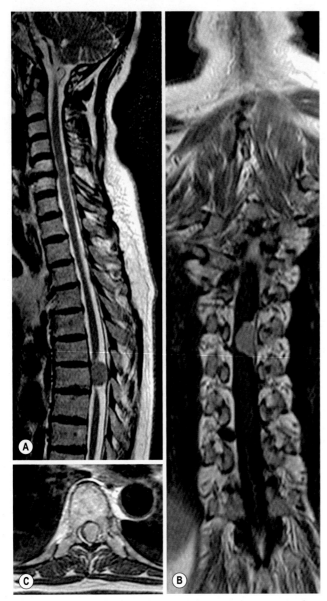

FIGURE 3-19 ■ **Mid-thoracic meningioma.** Sagittal T$_2$ (A) demonstrates an ovoid intradural extramedullary mass at the Th7 level. The lesion is slightly hyperintense relative to the spinal cord. Coronal (B) and axial (C) gadolinium-enhanced T$_1$ show avid contrast enhancement. Note the broad attachment to the dura with the presence of a typical dural tail. The tumour causes severe spinal canal narrowing and spinal cord compression and right lateral displacement of the spinal cord.

spinal cord and nerve roots, hence the name 'sugar coating' pattern; (2) multiple small contrast-enhancing nodules in the subarachnoid space (Fig. 3-21B); and (3) as a single contrast-enhancing mass.[4] However, sometimes metastases may not enhance, and careful inspection of T$_2$ or myelographic sequences is needed (Fig. 3-21C).

Less-Frequent Extramedullary Tumours

Less-frequent intradural, extramedullary tumours include paraganglioma, lipoma, epidermoid and dermoid cysts. In patients with von VHLs, intradural-extramedullary haemangioblastoma[30] and haemangioblastoma arising

from the proximal spinal nerve roots[47] have been described (Fig. 3-22).

Intradural Extramedullary Tumour Mimics

The differential diagnosis of intradural extramedullary tumours also include cysts and cyst-like lesions (arachnoid cysts, epidermoid and dermoid cysts, and teratoma, neuroenteric cysts), degenerative lesions (extruded disc fragment, discal cyst, juxtafacet cyst), inflammatory disorders affecting the nerve roots (Guillain–Barré syndrome, arachnoiditis, chronic interstitial demyelinating polyneuropathy (CIDP)) and, finally, infectious and granulomatous disorders (e.g. Lyme disease, sarcoidosis, Wegener's granulomatosis).[4]

Extradural Tumours

Extradural tumours are the most frequently observed spinal tumours; most of them originate from the vertebrae. Two-thirds of all spinal column lesions in children (<18) are benign, but this figure is reversed in adults.[48] Seventy-five per cent of vertebral body lesions are malignant, whereas benign lesions are mostly found in the posterior elements (70%).[48] Metastatic disease, multiple myeloma and lymphoproliferative tumours of the spine (e.g. lymphoma) commonly cause multiple lesions, which, in association with the clinical data, usually allow the diagnosis to be easily made. In contrast, the diagnosis of primary bone tumours must be considered when a solitary lesion is diagnosed.[2] Benign lesions are often asymptomatic and are frequently incidental findings on plain films realised, for example, after trauma. Pain was the most common presenting symptom, affecting 75% of the benign and 95% of the malignant tumours.[49] Extension of the tumour in the anterior epidural space displaces the lateral aspect of the posterior longitudinal ligament. However, this is limited by a strong medial fixation by the medial meningovertebral ligament (ligament of Trolard–Hofmann), giving a bilobular intracanalar aspect in the axial images, which is commonly called 'curtain sign' or 'draped curtain sign'. It may be observed in a variety of spinal tumours (Figs. 3-2, 3-23, 3-25, 3-38, and 3-39), both benign and malignant (Figs. 3-24–3-39), as well in other non-tumoural conditions such as epidural haematoma, epidural and abscesses. Epidural extension of the tumour may cause compression of the spinal cord or cauda equina with (progressive) paraplegia, saddle anaesthesia, urinary retention, incontinence and sexual dysfunction.

A multi-technique approach (CT, MR imaging, bone scintigraphy, PET) is often necessary to define the characteristics and extent of extradural spine neoplasms and bone scintigraphy is useful in detecting multiple lesions and distant metastases.[48] Because of the complex anatomy of the vertebrae, CT is more useful than plain film radiography for evaluating lesion location and analysing bone destruction, sclerosis and/or remodelling.[6] A wide variety of tumours that affect the bony spine may be encountered. It is possible to characterise these lesions based on the age of the patient, multiplicity, level in the spine and location within the vertebra. The differential

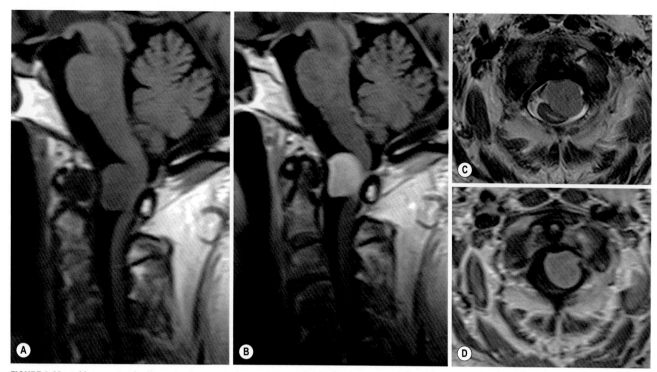

FIGURE 3-20 ■ **Upper cervical meningioma.** Sagittal T_1 (A) and gadolinium-enhanced T_1 (B) show an ovoid intradural extramedullary mass anteriorly in the spinal canal. The lesion is slightly hypointense when compared to the spinal cord and shows intense and homogeneous enhancement. A broad dural attachment can be observed. Compression and posterolateral displacement of the upper cervical cord by the tumour can be seen on the axial T_2 (C) and gadolinium-enhanced T_1 (D). A discrete area of high signal intensity on the axial T_2 can be seen, indicative of spinal cord oedema or compressive myelomalacia.

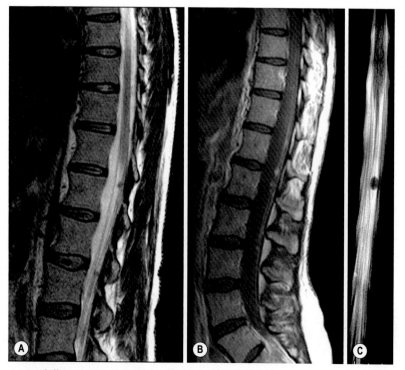

FIGURE 3-21 ■ **Intradural extramedullary metastases in a young woman with aggressive cervical cancer.** Sagittal T_2 (A) and sagittal gadolinium-enhanced T_1 (B) MR myelography (C). Nodular enhancing lesions along the nerve roots of the cauda equina are observed. Without proper clinical information, these lesions are indiscernible from multiple schwannomas as typically encountered in patients with NF-2 (see Fig. 3-17).

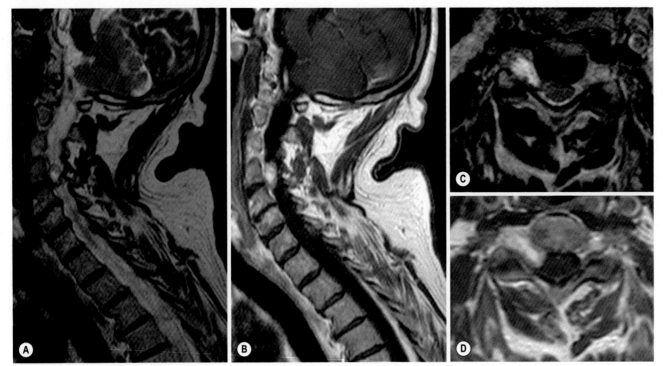

FIGURE 3-22 ■ Haemangioblastoma arising from the right C6 nerve in a patient with VHL syndrome. Sagittal T₂ (A) and contrast-enhanced T₁ (B) show the presence of a mass lesion laterally within the spinal canal. Intense enhancement of the lesion is observed. On axial T₂ (C) and Gd-enhanced T₁ (D), the lesion is arising from the right C6 proximal nerve root and can be classified as a combined intradural–extradural lesion, extending from the spinal canal towards the C5–C6 neuroforamen, which is enlarged.

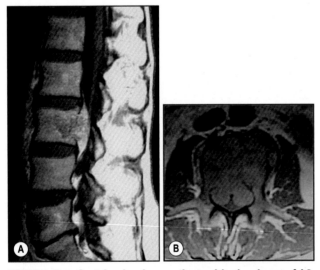

FIGURE 3-23 ■ Curtain sign in a patient with chordoma of L3. Sagittal (A) and axial (B) contrast-enhanced T₁ show a lesion located in the posterior aspect of the vertebral body with destruction of the posterior wall and extension into the anterior epidural space. A 'curtain sign' or 'draped curtain sign' is described whereby the midline is spared because of an intact ventral meningovertebral ligament, running from the anterior wall of the thecal sac to the posterior longitudinal ligament and vertebral endostium. These ligaments are significantly developed at the level of the conus and are known as the sacrodural ligaments of Trolard and Hofmann.

diagnosis can be further narrowed by evaluating the imaging findings, including morphology (border, matrix, expansion, soft-tissue involvement, etc.), density or signal intensity of lesions on CT and MR imaging, as well as pattern of contrast enhancement.[6]

Metastatic Spine Disease

Metastatic disease to the spine is the most frequent spinal tumour. Past or concurrent history of a primary tumour is generally available to suggest this diagnosis, but may need to be ascertained if the history is absent. Osteolytic metastases are most often caused by carcinoma of the lung, breast, thyroid, kidney and colon and (in childhood) neuroblastoma. Osteoblastic metastases are most commonly caused by prostate carcinoma in elderly men and by breast cancer in women. Metastasis to the spine most often involves the thoracic spine (70%), followed by the lumbar (20%) and cervical spine (10%). Multiple spinal levels are affected in about 30% of patients. Most frequently metastasis affects the vertebral body, but all parts of the vertebra may be affected. Vertebral compression fracture and epidural tumour extension are common in metastases.[2,6,48] Spinal metastases usually present as lytic lesions on plain film radiography, but one should keep in mind that metastatic disease is primarily a process of trabecular bone; plain film radiography is a cortical bone imaging technique. There must be 50 to 75% bone destruction for plain film radiographs to identify these lesions. On CT, metastatic disease presents as multiple lytic lesions of different size, with irregular non-sclerotic margins, often with cortical breakthrough

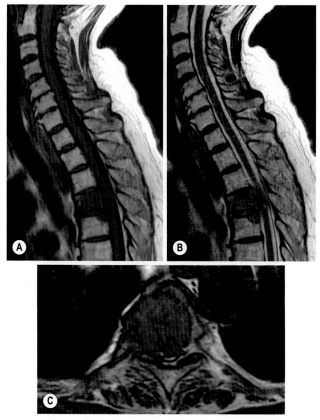

FIGURE 3-24 ■ **MR imaging shows osteoblastic metastatic disease in a woman with breast carcinoma.** Most metastases are hypointense on the sagittal T_1 (A) and when sclerotoc/osteoblastic they are also hypointense on T_2 (B). MRI better delineates the soft tissue extension of the tumour into the paraspinal and epidural soft tissues (C).

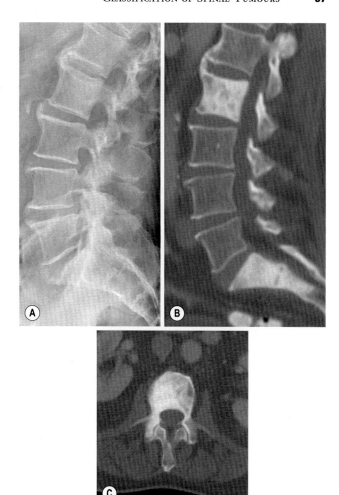

FIGURE 3-25 ■ **Metastatic spine disease in a patient with prostate carcinoma.** Lateral plain film radiography of the lumbar spine (A) shows a slight increased density of the L2 vertebral body. On sagittal (B) and axial (C) CT images, the lesion has the typical aspect of a 'ivory vertebra' due to the bony sclerosis. There is extension of the lesion in the right lateral pedicle. Additional osteoblastic metastases can be observed in S1 and S2.

and paravertebral or epidural extension. Osteoblastic metastases will show increased density and sclerosis and may have the aspect of an 'ivory vertebra' (Fig. 3-24). MR imaging is the preferred imaging technique in the evaluation of patients with suspected spinal metastasis. It allows imaging of the spine in one setting with greater sensitivity than bone imaging and delineates the soft-tissue extension of the tumour into the paraspinal and epidural soft tissues (Fig. 3-25C). On MR imaging most metastases are hypointense on T_1 (Fig. 3-25A). On T_2 they can be either dark (sclerotic) (Fig. 3-25B) or, more frequently, show high signal. Marked enhancement after contrast administration is the rule.

Primary Vertebral Tumours

Primary tumours of the vertebral column make up 10% of all spinal tumours and are rare compared with secondary malignancies. Primary vertebral tumours affect both the adult and the paediatric population and may be benign, locally aggressive, or malignant. Benign primary vertebral tumours include haemangioma, osteoid osteoma and osteoblastoma, aneurysmal bone cyst and eosinophilic granuloma. More locally aggressive primary vertebral tumours include chordoma and giant-cell tumour (GCT), whereas the most frequent malignant tumours are chondrosarcoma, Ewing's sarcoma, multiple myeloma

or plasmacytoma, and osteosarcoma.[50] In a review of the Leeds Regional Bone Tumour Registry for primary bone tumours of the spine (1958–2000), chordoma was the most frequent tumour in the cervical and sacral regions, while the most common diagnosis overall was multiple myeloma and plasmacytoma. Osteosarcoma ranked third.[49]

Benign Primary Vertebral Tumours

Vertebral Haemangioma

Vertebral haemangiomas are the most common benign spinal tumours, and the majority of lesions are discovered incidentally on spinal imaging performed for other purposes. In up to 30% of patients multiple lesions are observed. More than half of all vertebral haemangiomas are seen in the thoracic and lumbar spine. Most haemangiomas occur in the vertebral body, but about 10% may extend in the pedicles and even the spinous process may be involved. Two types of vertebral haemangioma exist: benign, asymptomatic lesions (Fig. 3-26), and more

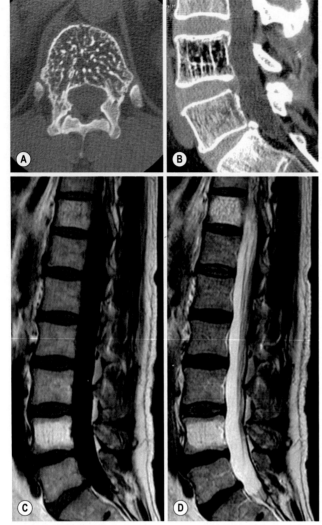

FIGURE 3-26 ■ **Asymptomatic vertebral haemangioma.** Axial CT (A) shows numerous high-attenuation dots within the vertebral bone marrow, simulating the 'polka-dot' pattern on clothing. On a sagittal reformatted image (B) a so-called 'corduroy sign' may be observed: vertically oriented, thickened trabeculations, replacing the normal cancellous bone, surrounded by fatty bone marrow or vascular lacunae. Sagittal T_1 (C) and T_2 (D) MR images show high (fat) signal intensity throughout the Th11 and L4 vertebral body with linear striations of low signal intensity due to thickened trabeculae.

aggressive, symptomatic ones, with compression of the spinal cord (Fig. 3-27).[6] Pregnancy may contribute to the development of aggressive and symptomatic haemangiomas, which is hypothesised to be caused by an increase in blood volume and cardiac output.[51]

The typical radiographic appearance of a haemangioma is characteristic, consisting of parallel linear streaks ('jail bar') in a vertebral body of overall decreased density, or 'honeycomb' pattern which may be also appreciated on sagittal reformatted images (Fig. 3-26B). Transverse CT shows the pattern as multiple dots, also known as 'polka-dot' pattern (Fig. 3-26A), representing a cross-section of reinforced trabeculae.[52] The key features that differentiate haemangiomas from other similar tumours are a hyperintense signal on T_1 (Fig. 3-26C) and T_2 (Fig. 3-26D).[51] The fibroadipose tissue insinuated between the

sinusoidal blood channels results in the increased T_1 signal pattern. These lesions will decrease in signal intensity on T_2 with fat saturation and will demonstrate contrast enhancement after gadolinium injection.[48] Low signal intensity on T_1 may indicate a more aggressive lesion with the potential to compress the spinal cord (Fig. 3-27A).[53] Aggressive lesions are characterised by a prominent soft-tissue component that can invade the epidural space and encroach on the spinal cord (Fig. 3-27).[48,54] The radiographic and CT appearances of compressive vertebral haemangiomas can be misleading, with irregular trabeculae and lytic areas; poorly defined, expanded cortex; and soft-tissue expansion.[2] Transarterial embolisation is an effective treatment for painful intraosseous haemangioma and is useful in reducing intraoperative blood loss before decompressive surgery.[55]

Osteoid Osteoma/Osteoblastoma

Osteoid osteomas (OOs) and osteoblastomas are histologically similar benign tumours consisting of osteoblasts that produce osteoid and woven bone.[56] OOs are smaller (less than 1.5 cm), well-contained, self-limited lesions, whereas osteoblastomas are larger (greater than 1.5 cm) and may undergo malignant transformation.[48] The peak incidence for OO is in the second decade. The average age at presentation is 17 years. Men are more affected than women (2–4 : 1). OO accounts for about 10% of all bone tumours involving the spine.[6] Almost 60% occur in the lumbar spine, 30% in the cervical spine and 10% in the thoracic spine. OO is a lesion of the posterior elements[57] with 50% of lesions arising in the lamina or pedicles and 20% in the articular processes.[48] Localised pain at the site of the lesion—classically worse at night—is the most common clinical presentation.[51] The pain is presumed to be caused by the presence of nerve endings in the nidus that are stimulated by vascular pressure and the production of prostaglandins, which explains the clinical response of these tumours to non-steroidal anti-inflammatory drugs (NSAIDs) such as aspirin.[48] Not infrequently, patients with spinal OO have a painful scoliosis.[6]

Plain film radiography may show a lucent nidus, frequently with small calcifications. Surrounding the nidus is variable bone sclerosis. The complex anatomy of the spine makes the detection and localisation of a radiolucent nidus obscured by reactive sclerosis much more difficult than that of a nidus located in a long bone.[2] Especially when there is extensive bone sclerosis, the nidus is much easier to distinguish on CT.[58] The nidus can be seen on CT as an area of low attenuation with various degrees of surrounding sclerosis (Fig. 3-28).[51] CT is the primary imaging technique used for diagnosis and to guide minimally invasive treatment such as interstitial laser ablation.[59] OOs can also be detected with MR imaging, with the nidus appearing as a hypointense lesion surrounded by marrow oedema on T_2. On T_1, the nidus can have an intermediate signal intensity and areas of signal voids resulting from calcification.[57] Enhancement within the nidus or perinidal marrow can be seen after gadolinium administration and can increase the sensitivity of the imaging study.[57]

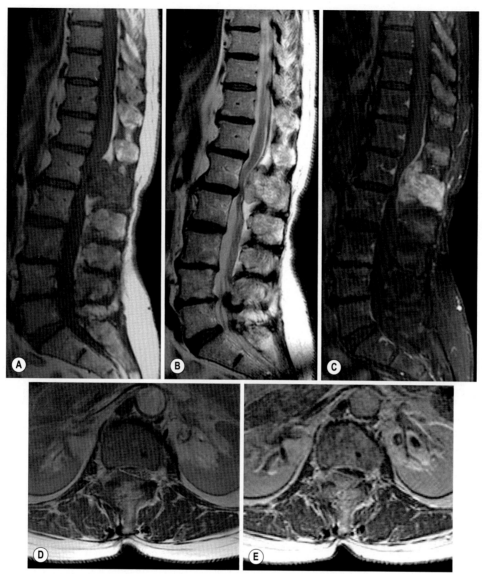

FIGURE 3-27 ■ **Aggressive variant of vertebral haemangioma.** Expansile lesion involving the posterior elements at the L1 level, leaving the pedicles and vertebral body intact. The lesion has low signal intensity on sagittal T_1 (A). Invasion of the posterior epidural space can be better evaluated on sagittal T_2 (B). Fat-suppressed gadolinium-enhanced T_1 (C) shows strong enhancement of the lesion. Axial T_2 (D) and gadolinium-enhanced T_1 (E) better show the mass effect of the tumour compressing the thecal sac, resulting in spinal stenosis with compression of the cauda equina.

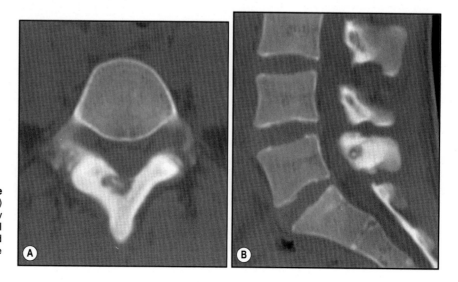

FIGURE 3-28 ■ **Osteoid osteoma of the posterior elements.** Axial CT image (A) and sagittal reformatted image (B) show a sclerotic bone lesion with a small central lucent nidus and dense calcified centre arising at the junction of the laminae of the L5 vertebra.

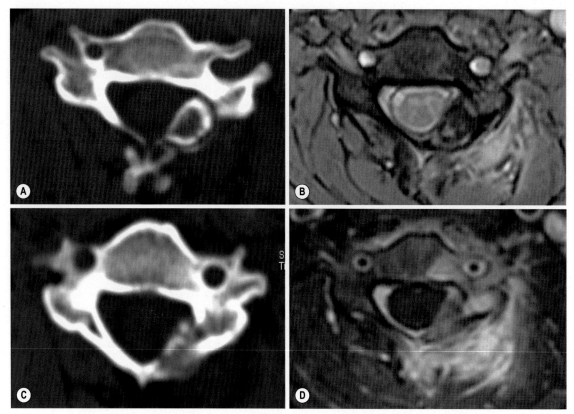

FIGURE 3-29 ■ **Osteoblastoma of the vertebral arch.** Axial CT images (A, B) demonstrate a partially calcified lesion at the left vertebral lamina. On axial T_1 (C) merely low signal intensity of the calcified lesion's component. Corresponding T_1 after contrast injection (D) shows marked contrast enhancement of the surrounding osseous and soft tissues.

Osteoblastoma

Osteblastomas are related to OOs, and by definition, are larger than 1.5 cm in diameter. They also have the tendency to affect the posterior part of the spine (Fig. 3-29) and present with pain. Osteoblastomas can be more aggressive than OOs and more often require surgical resection. The recurrency rate is about 10%, which is also higher than that seen with OOs.[6] Osteoblastoma has a similar appearance on CT, but displays less reactive sclerosis. The finding of central expansion similar to that of an aneurysmal bone cyst has also been described in spinal osteoblastoma.[51]

Aneurysmal Bone Cyst

Historically, aneurysmal bone cyst (ABC) was considered to be a variant of giant cell tumour (GCT). The microscopic appearances of the two lesions are sometimes strikingly similar, and they are occasionally indistinguishable.[60] Although ABC is classified as a primary bone tumour in many textbooks and scientific papers, Saccomanni states that ABC is a non-neoplastic reactive condition, which is aggressive in its ability to destroy and expand bone. The aetiology of an ABC is uncertain. It may occur in bone as a solitary lesion or can be found in association with other tumours such as GCT (Fig. 3-1) and chondroblastoma.[61] After osteoid osteoma and osteoblastoma, ABC is the third most frequent benign bone tumour.[62] Approximately 20 to 35% of ABC occur in the

spine, and ABCs represent 15% of all primary spine tumours.[63]

They afflict predominantly children, with 60% of patients being younger than 20 years.[61] The peak incidence is during the second decade of life, and they are slightly more common in female individuals.[64] They have a predilection for the lumbar spine, followed by equal occurrence in the thoracic and cervical spine. Of aneurysmal bone cysts, 60% occur in the pedicles, laminae and spinous processes;[61] however, the lesions can involve all aspects of the vertebrae, including the vertebral body. Clinical presentation includes pain, neurological deficit, and often scoliosis or kyphosis.[63]

Four radiological stages have been described by Kransdorf et al.: initial, active, stabilisation and healing.[60] In the initial phase, the lesion is characterised by a well-defined area of osteolysis. This is followed by a growth phase, in which the lesion has a purely lytic pattern and sometimes ill-defined margins. Later, during the stabilisation phase, the characteristic soap bubble appearance develops as a result of maturation of the bony shell.[60] The CT appearance of aneurysmal bone cysts is that of a ballooning, multilobulated lytic lesion that resembles a 'soap bubble' with a 'blown-out' appearance (Figs. 3-1B and D).[65] In a series by Hudson, 35% of ABCs showed fluid–fluid levels at CT.[66] Fluid–fluid levels within ABCs are indicative of haemorrhage with sedimentation and are better demonstrated with MR imaging (Fig. 3-30). On T_1, they may have increased signal intensity due to methaemoglobin in either the dependent or non-dependent

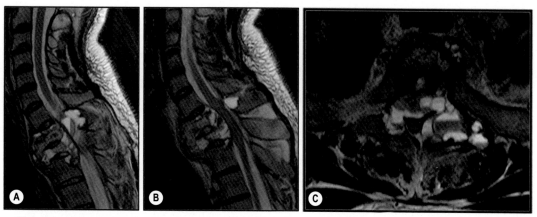

FIGURE 3-30 ■ **Aneurysmal bone cyst.** Sagittal (A, B) and axial (C) T_2 show an expansile process involving several segments of two thoracic vertebrae. Extension toward the spinal canal with spinal cord compression is observed. Presence of multiple fluid–fluid levels proves the haemorrhagic content of the lesions.

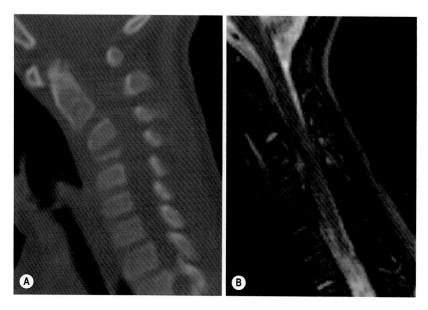

FIGURE 3-31 ■ **Eosinophilic granuloma in a 6-year-old girl with Langerhans cell histiocytosis.** Sagittal CT reformat of the C-spine (A) shows marked C4 vertebral compression ("vertebra plana") with kyphosis. Sagittal T2-weighted imaging (B) demonstrates intact vertebral endplates and adjacent disk spaces. A hyperintense soft tissue mass extending in the prevertebral tissues and anterior epidural space is observed. (Case courtesy of C. Venstermans, Antwerp, Belgium.)

component.[65] This finding is, however, not specific for ABCs, as it is also seen in other bone lesions, which contain areas of haemorrhage or necrosis such as telangiectatic osteosarcoma, GCT and chondroblastoma.[62] The lobulated lesion is surrounded by a hypointense rim on MR imaging corresponding to the intact periosteum or pseudocapsule.[65] The cystic components vary in appearance on T_1 and T_2, which is thought to represent the varying ages of the accumulated haemorrhage products within the cavities. Gadolinium enhancement is seen in up to 96% of lesions (Fig. 3-1E).[51] Peritumoural oedema is best defined on T_2 and STIR.[48] Although CT and MR imaging are diagnostic methods for many cases, it is noted in the literature that biopsy is necessary for confirmation, since many bone lesions can have a similar appearance.[61]

Eosinophilic Granuloma

Eosinophilic granuloma is a rare, benign solitary bone lesion that affects primarily children.[67] The peak incidence for eosinophilic granuloma of the spine is in the first decade. There is a clear male predilection.[6] Eosinophilic granuloma is one of the three clinical presentations of the disorder called Langerhans cell histiocytosis, formerly known as histiocytosis X, which can involve the central nervous system, bone, liver, lungs and lymph nodes. The most frequent sites of skeletal lesions are the skull, femur, mandible, pelvis and spine (least common).[68] In patients with Langerhans cell histiocytosis, the classic presentation of the vertebral lesions is that of vertebra plana, sometimes called 'pancake vertebra' on plain films (Fig. 3-31A).[68] There is a predilection for the thoracic spine, followed by the lumbar and then cervical spine. Vertebral bodies and anterior elements are involved much more commonly than the posterior elements. Lesions may be single or multiple. Eosinophilic granuloma has a highly variable clinical presentation, ranging from non-existent to very painful, sometimes worsening at night and sensitive to salicylate drugs or NSAIDs. The presenting symptoms of cervical eosinophilic granuloma are usually pain and restricted range of motion. In contrast to eosinophilic granuloma of the thoracic spine and lumbar spine, the neurological symptoms are less frequent.

Plain film radiography shows a lytic lesion with sharp borders. It is a classic cause of a single collapsed vertebral body (vertebra plana).[6] Nevertheless, vertebra plana is a rare sign in cervical eosinophilic granuloma.[67] If vertebral collapse is not complete, anterior wedging of the body may be observed. Mild epidural or soft-tissue extension may be seen on CT or MR imaging. Eosinophilic granuloma is isointense on T_1 and hyperintense on T_2. It enhances strongly with gadolinium. There is usually complete preservation of the adjacent discs (Fig. 3-31B). Vertebra plana in children can also occur as a result of a variety of malignant tumours, including Ewing's sarcoma, osteosarcoma and lymphomas. The wide differential diagnoses highlight the necessity for a thorough work-up, usually including an open, CT- or fluoroscopy-guided biopsy.[51,68]

Benign Notochordal Cell Tumours

Benign notochordal cell tumours (BNCTs) are benign tumours arising from embryonic remnants of the notochord, the midline craniocaudal cord of tissue involved in induction of the spine during embryogenesis, which subsequently involutes leaving normal remnants, the nucleus pulposus and abnormal remnants that can persist in adults along the spine.[69] They are found in approximately 20% of autopsy cases.[70] Previously, these tumours have been reported with various nomenclatures including 'ecchordosis physaliphora vertebralis',[71] vertebral intra-osseous chordoma,[72] giant notochordal rest,[72] giant notochordal hamartoma of intraosseous origin[73] and benign chordoma.[74] BNCTs are considered the benign counterpart of chordoma and are now described as a distinct entity, since clinically and histopathologically they lack characteristic features of chordomas and embryonic notochordal remnants.[74,75] However, these lesions may be precursors of chordoma.[74] Some authors hypothesise the existence of

a disease continuum from BNCT to incipient and then classic chordoma, as different stages of the same condition.[76] It is conceivable that pre-existing intraosseous BNCTs transform into incipient chordoma (Fig. 3-32) and then extend through the cortex into the surrounding soft tissue. This so-called 'incipient chordoma' has intermediate features between BNCT and chordoma. Histologically, they have the typical features of BNCT, but clinically they tend to behave like aggressive lesions, with osteolysis and extension of the tumour in the adjacent soft tissues.[70] BNCTs should be recognised by radiologists, pathologists and orthopaedic surgeons to prevent unnecessary radical surgery; on the other hand, close follow-up by cross-sectional imaging techniques is necessary to detect incipient lesions early, as they should be treated in the same manner as a classic chordoma.[76]

BNCTs are usually asymptomatic; mild pain is the most common symptom.[74] Most lesions (almost 75%) that are clinically identified arise in the mobile spine, typically the lumbar and cervical regions.[74] A series of seven cases arising from the posterior clivus have been published recently. Radiographic findings may be normal, or may show ill-defined, vague sclerosis within the vertebral body. More rarely, a diffuse prominent sclerosis presenting as ivory vertebra may be seen. Technetium bone scintigraphy show no abnormal uptake. On CT, BNCTs are typically sclerotic, and may replace the entire bone marrow of the vertebral body; cortical disruption or bone destruction are absent.[74] On MRI, BNCTs show a homogeneous low signal intensity on T_1 (Fig. 3-32A) and a homogeneous intermediate-to-high signal intensity on T_2 (Fig. 3-32B).[74] In a retrospective study of 38 patients with histopathological diagnosis of chordomas, Nishiguchi et al. noticed the absence of enhancement on contrast-enhanced series in BNCTs; all chordomas showed some degree of enhancement (Fig. 3-32C).[75] The most important discriminating feature between these two entities is the absence of a soft-tissue component in BNCTs, whereas the presence of a soft-tissue mass should indicate the diagnosis of chordoma.[74]

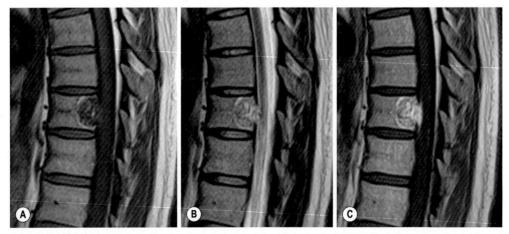

FIGURE 3-32 ■ **Follow-up MR examination of a benign notochordal cell tumour (BNCT)-incipient chordoma found initially as an incidental finding in a patient with a motor vehicle accident.** Sagittal T_1 (A) shows a geographic, sclerotic hypointense lesion with a discrete hyperintense rim. On sagittal T_2 (B) the lesion is displayed with high signal intensity. The enhancement of the lesion and the extension in the anterior epidural space on the gadolinium-enhanced T_1 (C) suggest transformation of a pre-existing intraosseous BNCT into incipient chordoma.

Locally Aggressive Primary Vertebral Tumours

Chordoma. Chordomas are the most common primary bone tumour of the sacrum and mobile spine.[49] Chordomas are exclusively observed in the spine, with two sites of predilection situated at the two extremities of the spine, the sacrum (50%)[77] (Fig. 3-33) and the skull base (35%).[69] The cervical location is the most commonly involved segment in the mobile spine (Fig. 3-34).[78,79] Chordomas were previously believed to arise from embryonic remnants of the notochord. However, recent studies suggest the possibility that chordomas arise from BNCTs.[70] The peak incidence for chordoma is between 50 and 60 years of age. Men are more affected than women.[80] Chordomas are considered low-grade, slow-growing, locally aggressive lesions.[80,81] Despite the lesion's slow expansion rate, the tumour is often quite large when first discovered, which results in difficulties in the surgical treatment and sometimes leads to a high local recurrence rate and a poor survival rate.[82] Although chordomas are not typically metastatic on presentation, the often late-stage diagnosis of the disease makes distant metastasis more likely. Five per cent of chordomas show metastasis to the lungs, bone, skin and brain at the time of initial presentation, and as high as 65% are metastatic in very advanced disease.[80] Accurate preoperative assessment is important in successful surgical resection with better prognosis.

Chordomas are midline lesions and often appear radiographically as destructive bone lesions, with an epicentre in the vertebral body and a surrounding soft-tissue mass. On CT, an expansive, midline lytic lesion with irregular borders and infiltration of surrounding tissues is observed. Calcification and bone sclerosis are frequently present. Paravertebral and epidural extension of the lesion can be evaluated.[83] Because of the variety of components, most lesions are heterogeneous on MR imaging. The most striking feature of a chordoma is the high signal intensity seen on T_2 (Figs. 3-33B and 3-33E).

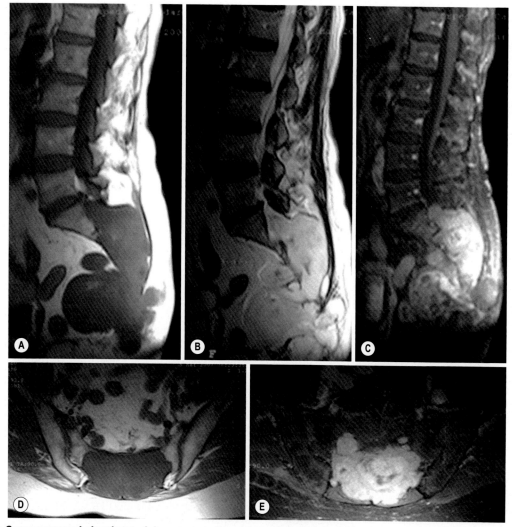

FIGURE 3-33 ■ **Sacrococcygeal chordoma.** A large expansile and multilobulated midline tumour with extensive anterior soft-tissue involvement is found. The tumour looks well-encapsulated, and some internal septations can be seen. The tumour displays rather homogeneous low signal intensity on sagittal T_1 (A) and homogeneous high signal intensity on T_2 (B). Sagittal fat-suppressed contrast-enhanced T_1 (C) reveals heterogeneous enhancement throughout the mass. Axial T_2 (D) and fat-suppressed contrast-enhanced T_1 (E) show non-involvement of the sacroiliac joints. (Case courtesy of M. Thurnher, Vienna, Austria.)

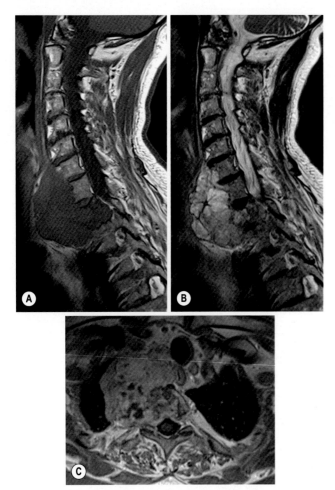

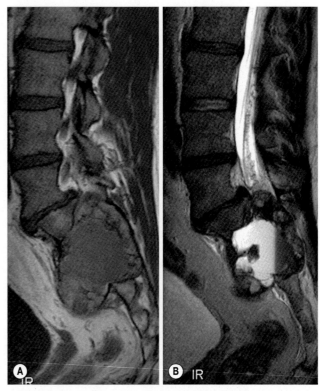

FIGURE 3-35 ■ **Giant cell tumour from the sacrum.** Heterogeneous expansile tumour arising at the S1–S2 level. Low signal intensity components at the periphery of the lesion on both sagittal T_1 (A) and T_2 (B). Large fluid–fluid level with low signal intensity of the dependent part due to sedimentation of blood components on T_2-weighted image.

FIGURE 3-34 ■ **Chordoma of the mobile spine.** Sagittal T_1 (A), and sagittal T_2-weighted images and axial T_1 image after Gd injection (C) show a polylobular lesion originating at the body of Th1 and extending anteriorly, invading the anterior aspect of the C6 and C7 vertebral bodies. The lesion is of intermediate signal intensity on T_1 (A) and has mixed, intermediate and high signal intensity on T_2 (B). There is marked, non-homogeneous contrast enhancement of both the osseous and soft-tissue component of the tumour (C).

This is due to abundant intra- and extracellular mucin produced by the tumour.[84] Chordomas tend to show hypointense or isointense signal relative to that of muscle on T_1 (Fig. 3-33A). Areas of hyperintensity on T_1 typically represent areas of haemorrhage or high protein content of the myxoid and mucinous collections.[77,84] The presence of haemosiderin in chordomas accounts for the low signal intensity seen with T_2.[84] The pattern of enhancement after gadolinium injection can be variable (Fig. 3-33C), ranging from homogeneous to peripheral septal enhancement.[50] The septal pattern is presumably produced by the presence of chondroid tissues or the degree of the lobules with mucogelatinous contents of these tumours.[84] Chordomas arising in the mobile spine typically show a soft-tissue mass spanning several vertebral segments (Fig. 3-34). Most of the lesions show a so-called 'collar button' appearance on sagittal images. Cervical chordomas display a 'dumbbell' morphology or 'mushroom' appearance without bone involvement and with enlargement of the neuroforamen mimicking a neurogenic tumour.[78] The combination of high signal on T_2

and a lobulated sacral mass that contains areas of haemorrhage and calcification is strongly suggestive of a chordoma.[77]

Giant Cell Tumours. Giant cell tumours (GCTs) involving the spine are rare (7%).[85] They occur in skeletally mature patients in the second to fourth decades of life, more frequently in females.[2] Ten to 15% may have an ABC-like component (Fig. 3-1).[48] Most of these lesions occur in the sacrum, followed in order of decreasing frequency by the thoracic, cervical and lumbar segments of the mobile spine.[85] GCTs are the second most common primary bone tumour of the sacrum (after chordomas), usually located in the upper part of the sacrum and frequently lateralised in a sacral wing (Fig. 3-35).[50] Extension to the iliac wing through the sacroiliac joint is possible.[2] Unlike most benign tumours of the spine, GCTs are found in greater frequency in the vertebral body (55%) but often involve the body and posterior elements (30%).[48] Extraosseous involvement of the soft tissues is seen in 79% of cases.[2] A dramatic increase in lesion size can occasionally be associated with pregnancy and is presumably related to hormonal stimulation.[85]

Plain film radiography demonstrates a well-demarcated lytic and expansile lesion that often crosses the midline in the sacrum and may cross the sacroiliac joints. There is typically a narrow zone of transition.[85] CT better defines the characteristics identified on plain film images and better defines the bone architecture of the lesion. CT demonstrates absence of mineralisation and the lack of a

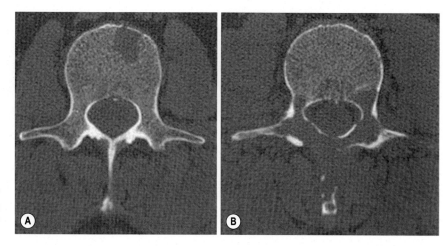

FIGURE 3-36 ■ Multiple myeloma. CT (A, B) shows purely osteolytic lesions in different parts of several vertebrae and in the sacrum.

sclerotic rim at the margins of the tumour. MR imaging characteristics can be helpful in the diagnosis. A low-to-intermediate signal intensity on T_2 (Fig. 3-35B) is often seen within the lesion, which is thought to be secondary to the relative collagen content of fibrous components and haemosiderin within the lesion.[86] The tumour usually has low-to-intermediate signal intensity on T_1 (Fig. 3-35A). These lesions may also demonstrate curvilinear areas of low signal intensity on T_1 and T_2, which may correspond to thickened trabeculae or fibrous septae.[85] Enhancement of the lesion reflects its vascular supply. Cystic areas, foci of haemorrhage, fluid–fluid levels and a peripheral low-signal-intensity pseudocapsule may also be seen.[87,88]

Primary Malignant Vertebral Tumours

In the Leeds Regional Bone Tumour Registry, which focuses on spine tumours, primary malignant tumours of the spine constituted only 4.6% of the cases registered between 1958 and 2000.[49] The most common malignant spine tumours were multiple myeloma and plasmacytoma. The second most common tumour was chordoma. The third most common tumour was osteosarcoma.[89]

Multiple Myeloma and Plasmacytoma

Multiple myeloma and plasmacytoma are the most common malignant vertebral tumours.[49] Multiple myeloma is a disease of infiltrative plasma B cells that can spread to the mobile spine and sacrum. In approximately 5% of patients, the disease may manifest as a solitary plasmacytoma of bone, with a frequent site of presentation being the spine. Two-thirds of these patients have been reported to go on to develop multiple myeloma.[48,89] These lesions occur twice as commonly in men as in women and have peak incidence at approximately 55 years of age. They have a preference for the thoracic spine. The vertebral body is the most common site of involvement because of its rich red marrow content, but the tumour frequently extends to the pedicles (Fig. 3-36B);[87] also epidural extension is a frequent finding. Multiple areas of spinal involvement frequently result in pain and multiple compression fractures with the potential for collapse, spinal instability and neurological deficit from spinal cord compression.

In two-thirds of cases, plain film radiography will show plasmacytoma as a lytic and usually expansile bone lesion with thickened trabeculae and multicystic appearance.[6,87] The tumour preferentially replaces the cancellous bone, whereas the cortical bone is partly preserved or even sclerotic, resulting in a hollow vertebral body or pedicle on CT images (Fig. 3-36). In one-third of cases, the radiographic appearance is less characteristic, with a multicystic 'soap bubble' appearance simulating a haemangioma.[2,87] Plasmacytoma shows low signal intensity on T_1, high signal intensity on T_2 and homogeneous vivid enhancement on post-contrast T_1.[87,90] Curvilinear low-signal-intensity structures extending partially through the vertebral body and resembling sulci seen in the brain, causing a 'mini brain' appearance on axial images, have been described to be typical.[90] These low-signal-intensity structures are likely caused by thickened cortical bone caused by the slow-growing nature of plasmacytoma. This appearance can also be seen on CT. Focal end-plate fractures are well described in patients with plasmacytoma.[91] Involvement of the intervertebral disc and adjacent vertebrae can be used to help differentiate plasmacytoma from metastasis.[2,91]

In patients with multiple myeloma, imaging typically reveals diffuse lytic, 'punched-out' lesions within single or multiple vertebrae (Fig. 3-37). In some cases, there may be no characteristic findings. Diffuse osteoporosis of the vertebral bodies or multiple compression fractures may be observed.[50] Even in advanced stages of this disease, up to 20% of plain films and MR imaging studies may show normal findings. MDCT allows imaging of the entire spine and provides detailed information on osseous involvement in multiple myeloma.[92] Especially in anatomically complex regions such as the pelvis and the thoracic spine, it is superior to plain film radiography. Compared with conventional radiography and MR imaging, MDCT provides more detailed information on the risk of vertebral fractures.[93] For evaluating diffuse bone marrow changes, MR imaging is still the imaging technique of choice. Different signal patterns may be observed, ranging from normal-appearing bone marrow to focal lesions or diffuse bone marrow infiltration. On T_1, a low signal intensity is typically noted (Fig. 3-37A), with marked enhancement after the administration of gadolinium. Lesion conspicuity is increased on T_2 by using fat saturation or STIR techniques (Figs. 3-37B vs

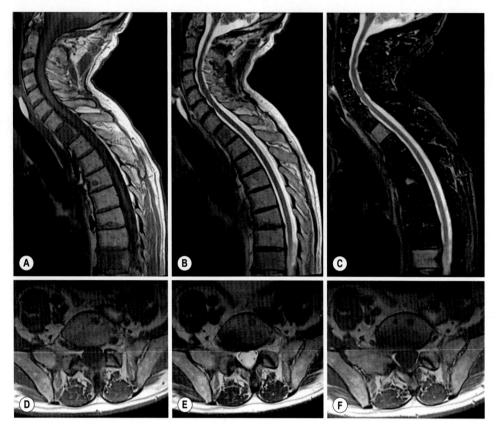

FIGURE 3-37 ▪ **Multiple mye-loma.** Sagittal T1 (A), sagittal T2 (B), and sagittal fat-supressed T2 (STIR) (C) and axial T1 (D), axial T2 (E) and axial contrast-enhanced T1-wi (F) reveal lytic, 'punched-out' lesions in the Th4 vertebral body and sacrum. Diffuse bone marrow involve-ment of Th1 and Th8 vertebral bodies is observed with replace-ment of the normal fatty bone marrow by low to intermediate signal intensity on T1 and T2. The lesions show marked high signal intensity on STIR.

C). Also T_1 completed after contrast administration should include fat saturation. Focal myeloma lesions in the spine may look similar to metastatic lesions on MR imaging, with pathological fracture, marrow replacement and epidural spread of the tumour.[48]

Chondrosarcoma

The most prevalent types of sarcomas involving the spine are chondrosarcoma, osteosarcoma, and Ewing's sarcoma.[89] Chondrosarcoma is the second most common non-myeloproliferative primary malignant tumour of the spine in adults.[65] Chondrosarcoma is a malignant tumour in which the basic neoplastic tissue is fully developed cartilage without tumour osteoid being directly formed by a sarcomatous stroma. Myxoid changes, calcification or ossification may be present.[89] Chondrosarcomas compose 7 to 12% of all primary spine tumours and account for up to 25% of malignant spine tumours. Men are affected 2 to 4 times more frequently than women; mean age of patients is 45 years. The thoracic and lumbar spine are most frequently affected, with the sacrum being affected only rarely.[94] Chondrosarcoma originates in the vertebral body (15% of cases), posterior elements (40%) or both (45%).[2] Chondrosarcomas of the spine are usually low-grade (either grade 1 or 2) lesions that may arise de novo as primary malignant tumours or as secondary transformations of osteochondromas or Paget's disease.

Although plain films may identify bone destruction and chondroid mineralisation in up to 70% of cases, cross-sectional imaging, including CT and MR imaging in combination, offers the best opportunity to define the tumour matrix and tumour extent (Figs. 3-2 and

3-38).[48] Chondrosarcomas of the spine usually manifest as a large, calcified mass with bone destruction.[95,96] True ossification may be seen, which corresponds to residual osteochondroma in cases of secondary chondrosarcoma.[87] Chondroid matrix mineralisation is better demonstrated with CT (Fig. 3-2C). Calcified matrix is detected as areas of signal void at MR imaging. The non-mineralised portion of the tumour has low attenuation on CT images, low-to-intermediate signal intensity on T_1 (Fig. 3-38A), and very high signal intensity on T_2 due to the high water content of hyaline cartilage (Figs. 3-38B and 3-38D). An enhancement pattern of 'rings and arcs' on gadolinium-enhanced images reflects the lobulated growth pattern of these cartilaginous tumours (Fig. 3-38E).[2]

Ewing's Sarcoma

Although the vertebral column is frequently involved in preterminal metastatic Ewing's sarcoma, primary vertebral Ewing's sarcoma is quite rare, with a reported prevalence of 3.5–15%.[97] Primary vertebral Ewing's sarcoma is usually seen in the second decade of life, with a slight male predilection. Ewing's sarcoma can involve all segments of the spine, with sacral involvement in as many as 50%.[97] The ala is the most frequently affected sacral site (69%); the majority (60%) of lesions in the mobile spine originate in the posterior elements with extension into the vertebral body.[97] Clinical presentation of Ewing's sarcoma is aspecific and includes pain and often neurological deficits.[50]

A permeative appearance that may mimic osteomyelitis is the hallmark of Ewing's tumour of the spine. This characteristic can be demonstrated on plain film

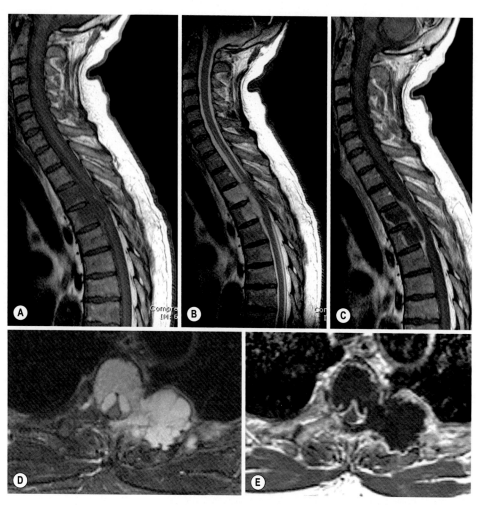

FIGURE 3-38 ■ **Chondrosarcoma.** Sagittal T1 (A), T2 (B) and contrast-enhanced T1 (C) show invasion of the Th3 and Th4 vertebral bodies with low-to-intermediate signal intensity on T1 and very high signal intensity on T2. Extension of the tumour in the anterior epidural space with spinal cord compression is observed. Peripheral irregular enhancement of the tumour. CT-guided percutaneous biopsy of the paravertebral extension of the tumour was performed (Fig. 3.2), and the final diagnosis of low-grade chondrosarcoma was made.

radiography, but CT has greater sensitivity.[98] Vertebra plana may be seen, and two or more adjacent vertebra may be involved. Fifty per cent of tumours have a non-calcified soft-tissue mass.[48] MRI is the imaging study of choice for local tumour staging. The MRI appearance can be extremely variable, depending on matrix formation and the degree of bone and soft-tissue involvement. Most often Ewing's sarcoma is iso- to hyperintense on T_2 (Fig. 3-39A) and isointense on T_1 (Fig. 3-39B and D). Contrast enhancement after gadolinium injection is seen because of the hypercellularity of the tumour (Fig. 3-39C and E).[50] Invasion of the spinal canal is frequent and the paraspinal component is often larger than the intraosseous lesion.[2] FDG-PET/CT is the new standard for initial staging and the detection of recurrence or new metastatic disease.[98] The initial standardised uptake value of the primary tumour has been shown to correlate with tumour aggressiveness.[48]

Osteosarcoma

Osteosarcoma is a high-grade malignant osteoblastic lesion. It is the third most common primary vertebral tumour. Primary vertebral osteosarcoma represents 4% of all osteosarcomas; secondary vertebral osteosarcoma may result from Paget's disease and radiation. Although osteosarcoma, overall, has a peak incidence during the adolescent growth spurt, spinal osteosarcoma tends to occur in an older age group, with a mean age of 38 years.[48] There is no sex- or race-based predilection.[89] Osteosarcoma can be found anywhere in the spine; the thoracic and lumbar segments are involved with equal frequency, followed by the sacrum and the cervical column.[99] In the mobile spine 80% of the lesions are found in the posterior elements with partial vertebral body involvement.[99] Other studies quote a significantly higher percentage of involvement of the vertebral body.[89] Most of the lesions occur at a single spinal segment but 17% involve more than one level. The clinical presentation of osteosarcoma is similar to that of Ewing's sarcoma: patients may present with pain, signs of neurological compression, or a palpable mass.[2] All osteosarcomas, despite their classification as to subtype (osteogenic, chondroblastic, fibroblastic, secondary osteosarcoma), have as their common feature the production of bone (osteoid) by neoplastic osteoblasts.[89]

A multi-technique approach to imaging is vital in defining the presence and extent of spine osteosarcoma. The variable pathological appearance, including osteoid matrix, marked mineralisation, ivory vertebrae, primary lytic pattern and a chondroblastic subtype, leads to a variety of imaging appearances.[99] Plain film radiography may demonstrate cortical destruction, a wide zone of transition, a permeative appearance or bone matrix. CT will better demonstrate these findings (Fig. 3-40) and is the best technique for defining matrix and bone

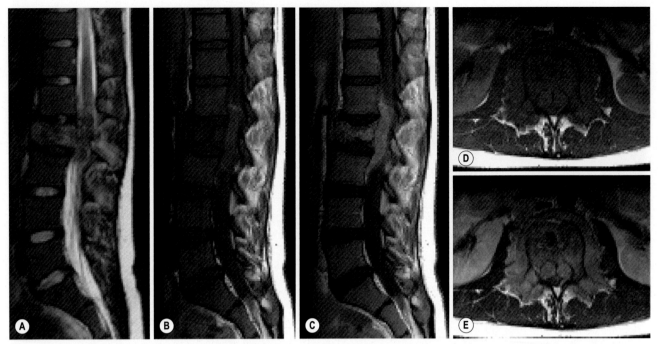

FIGURE 3-39 ■ **Ewing sarcoma of the L2 vertebral body.** The normal signal intensity of the fatty bone marrow is replaced and mild collapse of the vertebral body can be seen on the sagittal images. On the sagittal T2 (A), the lesion has a slight increased signal intensity. On the sagittal and axial T1 (B and D), the tumour is almost isointense and intense gadolinium-enhancement is observed (C and E). Invasion of the spinal canal ('curtain sign') and extension of the tumour in the adjacent paraspinal soft tissues is best demonstrated on the axial images.

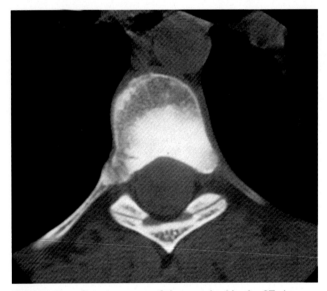

FIGURE 3-40 ■ **Osteosarcoma of the vertebral body.** CT shows a geographic, ill-defined, and non-expansile osteoblastic lesion in the posterior aspect of a thoracic vertebral body.

destruction.[48] Findings on MR imaging are extremely variable, with the signal abnormality based on the pathological subtype of the tumour.[89] Non-mineralised tumours will typically have a low signal on T_1 and high signal on T_2. Densely mineralised tumours, however, may demonstrate decreased signal on both T_1 and T_2. Gadolinium-enhanced images will better show the extension of the tumour in the surrounding soft tissues, particularly the intraspinal extension and the degree of central canal compromise. PET/CT is the current standard of care to stage all patients with bone and soft-tissue sarcomas. PET imaging is also used to monitor treatment response and conduct surveillance for recurrence.[48]

REFERENCES

1. Balériaux D, Parizel PM, Bank WO. Intraspinal and intramedullary pathology. In: Manelfe C, editor. Imaging of the Spine and Spinal Cord. New York: Raven Press; 1992. pp. 513–64.
2. Rodallec MH, Feydy A, Larousserie F, et al. Diagnostic imaging of solitary tumors of the spine: What to do and say. Radiographics 2008;28(4):1019–41.
3. De Beuckeleer L, van den Hauwe L, Bracke P, et al. Imaging of primary tumors and tumor-like conditions of the lumbosacral osseous spine. J Belge Radiol 1997;80(1):21–5.
4. Abul-Kasim K, Thurnher MM, McKeever P, Sundgren PC. Intradural spinal tumors: current classification and MRI features. Neuroradiology 2008;50(4):301–14.
5. Mechtler LL, Nandigam K. Spinal cord tumors. Neurol Clin 2013;31(1):241–68.
6. Van Goethem JWM, van den Hauwe L, Özsarlak Ö, et al. Spinal tumors. Eur J Radiol 2004;50(2):159–76.
7. Parizel PM, Balériaux D, Rodesch G, et al. Gd-DTPA-enhanced MR imaging of spinal tumors. Am J Roentgenol 1989;152(5):1087–96.
8. Balériaux DL. Spinal cord tumors. Eur Radiol 1999;9(7):1252–8.
9. Sugahara T, Korogi Y, Hirai T, et al. Contrast-enhanced T1-weighted three-dimensional gradient-echo MR imaging of the whole spine for intradural tumor dissemination. Am J Neuroradiol 1998;19(9):1773–9.
10. Thurnher MM, Law M. Diffusion-weighted imaging, diffusion-tensor imaging, and fiber tractography of the spinal cord. Magn Reson Imaging Clin N Am 2009;17(2):225–44.
11. Ducreux D, Fillard P, Facon D, et al. Diffusion tensor magnetic resonance imaging and fiber tracking in spinal cord lesions: current and future indications. Neuroimaging Clin N Am. 2007;17(1):137–47.
12. Vargas MI, Delavelle J, Jlassi H, et al. Clinical applications of diffusion tensor tractography of the spinal cord. Neuroradiology 2008;50(1):25–9.

13. Setzer M, Murtagh RD, Murtagh FR, et al. Diffusion tensor imaging tractography in patients with intramedullary tumors: comparison with intraoperative findings and value for prediction of tumor resectability. J Neurosurg Spine 2010;13(3):371–80.

14. Tomura N, Ito Y, Matsuoka H, et al. PET findings of intramedullary tumors of the spinal cord using [^{18}F] FDG and [^{11}C] methionine. Am J Neuroradiol 2013;34(6):1278–83.

15. Wilmshurst JM, Barrington SF, Pritchard D, et al. Positron emission tomography in imaging spinal cord tumors. J Child Neurol 2000;15(7):465–72.

16. Louis DN, Ohgaki H, Wiestler OD, et al. The 2007 WHO classification of tumours of the central nervous system. Acta Neuropathol 2007;114(2):97–109.

17. Chamberlain MC, Tredway TL. Adult primary intradural spinal cord tumors: a review. Curr Neurol Neurosci Rep 2011;11(3): 320–8.

18. Rossi A, Gandolfo C, Morana G, Tortori-Donati P. Tumors of the spine in children. Neuroimaging Clin N Am 2007;17(1): 17–35.

19. Koeller KK, Rosenblum RS, Morrison AL. Neoplasms of the spinal cord and filum terminale: radiologic-pathologic correlation. Radiographics 2000;20(6):1721–49.

20. Nemoto Y, Inoue Y, Tashiro T, et al. Intramedullary spinal cord tumors: significance of associated haemorrhage at MR imaging. Radiology 1992;182(3):793–6.

21. Smith AB, Soderlund KA, Rushing EJ, Smirniotopolous JG. Radiologic-pathologic correlation of pediatric and adolescent spinal neoplasms: Part 1, Intramedullary spinal neoplasms. Am J Roentgenol 2012;198(1):34–43.

22. Plotkin SR, O'Donnell CC, Curry WT, et al. Spinal ependymomas in neurofibromatosis Type 2: a retrospective analysis of 55 patients. J Neurosurg Spine 2011;14(4):543–7.

23. Khalatbari MR, Jalaeikhoo H, Hamidi M, Moharamzad Y. Craniospinal dissemination of filum myxopapillary ependymoma following spinal trauma: case report and literature review. Childs Nerv Syst 2013;29(1):149–52.

24. Brotchi J, Dewitte O, Levivier M, et al. A survey of 65 tumors within the spinal cord: surgical results and the importance of preoperative magnetic resonance imaging. Neurosurgery 1991;29(5):651–6, discussion 656–7.

25. Lee DK, Choe WJ, Chung CK, Kim H-J. Spinal cord hemangioblastoma: surgical strategy and clinical outcome. J Neurooncol 2003;61(1):27–34.

26. Baker KB, Moran CJ, Wippold FJ, et al. MR imaging of spinal hemangioblastoma. Am J Roentgenol 2000;174(2):377–82.

27. Lonser RR, Glenn GM, Walther M, et al. von Hippel-Lindau disease. Lancet 2003;361(9374):2059–67.

28. Takai K, Taniguchi M, Takahashi H, et al. Comparative analysis of spinal hemangioblastomas in sporadic disease and von Hippel-Lindau syndrome. Neurol Med Chir (Tokyo) 2010;50(7):560–7.

29. Wanebo JEJ, Lonser RRR, Glenn GMG, Oldfield EHE. The natural history of hemangioblastomas of the central nervous system in patients with von Hippel-Lindau disease. J Neurosurg 2002; 98(1):82–94.

30. Imagama S, Ito Z, Wakao N, et al. Differentiation of localization of spinal hemangioblastomas based on imaging and pathological findings. Eur Spine J 2011;20(8):1377–84.

31. Lonser RR, Vortmeyer AO, Butman JA, et al. Edema is a precursor to central nervous system peritumoral cyst formation. Ann Neurol 2005;58(3):392–9.

32. Chu BC, Terae S, Hida K, et al. MR findings in spinal hemangioblastoma: correlation with symptoms and with angiographic and surgical findings. Am J Neuroradiol 2001;189(6 Suppl):206–17. Available from: <http://eutils.ncbi.nlm.nih.gov/entrez/eutils/elink.fcgi?dbfrom=pubmed&id=18029903&retmode=ref&cmd=prlinks=>.

33. Patel UU, Pinto RSR, Miller DCD, et al. MR of spinal cord ganglioglioma. Am J Neuroradiol 1998;19(5):879–87.

34. Houten JKJ, Weiner HLH. Pediatric intramedullary spinal cord tumors: special considerations. J Neurooncol 2000;47(3): 225–30.

35. Castillo M. Gangliogliomas: ubiquitous or not? Am J Neuroradiol 1998;19(5):807–9.

36. Kalayci M, Cağavi F, Gül S, et al. Intramedullary spinal cord metastases: diagnosis and treatment—an illustrated review. Acta Neurochir 2004;146(12):1347–54, discussion 1354.

37. Rykken JB, Diehn FE, Hunt CH, et al. Rim and flame signs: postgadolinium MRI findings specific for non-CNS intramedullary spinal cord metastases. Am J Neuroradiol 2013;34(4):908–15.

38. Lee M, Epstein FJ, Rezai AR, Zagzag D. Nonneoplastic intramedullary spinal cord lesions mimicking tumors. Neurosurgery 1998; 43(4):788–94, discussion 794–5.

39. Hegde A, Mohan S, Tan KK, Lim CCT. Spinal cavernous malformations: magnetic resonance imaging and associated findings. Singapore Med J 2012;53(9):582–6.

40. Soderlund KA, Smith AB, Rushing EJ, Smirniotopolous JG. Radiologic-pathologic correlation of pediatric and adolescent spinal neoplasms: Part 2, Intradural extramedullary spinal neoplasms. Am J Roentgenol 2012;198(1):44–51.

41. Mautner VF, Tatagiba M, Lindenau M, et al. Spinal tumors in patients with neurofibromatosis type 2: MR imaging study of frequency, multiplicity, and variety. Am J Roentgenol 1995;165(4): 951–5.

42. De Verdelhan O, Haegelen C, Carsin-Nicol B, et al. MR imaging features of spinal schwannomas and meningiomas. J Neuroradiol 2005;32(1):42–9.

43. Wippold FJ, Smirniotopoulos JG, Moran CJ, et al. MR imaging of myxopapillary ependymoma: findings and value to determine extent of tumor and its relation to intraspinal structures. Am J Roentgenol 1995;165(5):1263–7.

44. Ando K, Imagama S, Ito Z, et al. Differentiation of spinal schwannomas and myxopapillary ependymomas: MR imaging and pathologic features. J Spinal Disord Tech [Epub ahead of print]. 2012;

45. Freilich RJ, Krol G, DeAngelis LM. Neuroimaging and cerebrospinal fluid cytology in the diagnosis of leptomeningeal metastasis. Ann Neurol 1995;38(1):51–7.

46. Yuh EL, Barkovich AJ, Gupta N. Imaging of ependymomas: MRI and CT. Childs Nerv Syst 2009;25(10):1203–13.

47. Escott EJ, Kleinschmidt-Demasters BK, Brega K, Lillehei KO. Proximal nerve root spinal hemangioblastomas: presentation of three cases, MR appearance, and literature review. Surg Neurol 2004;61(3):262–73, discussion 273.

48. Wald JT. Imaging of spine neoplasm. Radiol Clin North Am 2012;50(4):749–76.

49. Kelley SP, Ashford RU, Rao AS, Dickson RA. Primary bone tumours of the spine: a 42-year survey from the Leeds Regional Bone Tumour Registry. Eur Spine J 2007;16(3):405–9.

50. Ropper AE, Cahill KS, Hanna JW, et al. Primary vertebral tumors: a review of epidemiologic, histological and imaging findings, part II: locally aggressive and malignant tumors. Neurosurgery 2012; 70(1):211–9, discussion 219.

51. Ropper AE, Cahill KS, Hanna JW, et al. Primary vertebral tumors: a review of epidemiologic, histological, and imaging findings, Part I: benign tumors. Neurosurgery 2011;69(6):1171–80.

52. Ross JS, Masaryk TJ, Modic MT, et al. Vertebral hemangiomas: MR imaging. Radiology 1987;165(1):165–9.

53. Laredo JD, Assouline E, Gelbert F, et al. Vertebral hemangiomas: fat content as a sign of aggressiveness. Radiology 1990;177(2): 467–72.

54. Karaeminogullari O, Tuncay C, Demirors H, et al. Multilevel vertebral hemangiomas: two episodes of spinal cord compression at separate levels 10 years apart. Eur Spine J 2005;14(7):706–10.

55. Cross JJ, Antoun NM, Laing RJ, Xuereb J. Imaging of compressive vertebral haemangiomas. Eur Radiol 2000;10(6):997–1002.

56. Kan P, Schmidt MH. Osteoid osteoma and osteoblastoma of the spine. Neurosurg Clin N Am 2008;19(1):65–70.

57. Harish S, Saifuddin A. Imaging features of spinal osteoid osteoma with emphasis on MRI findings. Eur Radiol. 2005;15(12):2396–403. Available from: <http://eutils.ncbi.nlm.nih.gov/entrez/eutils/elink.fcgi?dbfrom=pubmed&id=15973540&retmode=ref&cmd=prlinks=>.

58. Youssef BA, Haddad MC, Zahrani A, et al. Osteoid osteoma and osteoblastoma: MRI appearances and the significance of ring enhancement. Eur Radiol 1996;6(3):291–6.

59. Gangi A, Alizadeh H, Wong L, et al. Osteoid osteoma: percutaneous laser ablation and follow-up in 114 patients. Radiology 2007;242(1):293–301.

60. Kransdorf MJM, Sweet DED. Aneurysmal bone cyst: concept, controversy, clinical presentation, and imaging. Am J Roentgenol 1995;164(3):573–80.

61. Saccomanni B. Aneurysmal bone cyst of spine: a review of literature. Arch Orthop Trauma Surg 2008;128(10):1145–7.

62. Zileli M, Isik HS, Ogut FE, et al. Aneurysmal bone cysts of the spine. Eur Spine J 2013;22(3):593–601.

63. Boriani SS, De Iure FF, Campanacci LL, et al. Aneurysmal bone cyst of the mobile spine: report on 41 cases. Spine 2000;26(1):27–35.

64. Mankin HJ, Hornicek FJ, Ortiz-Cruz E, et al. Aneurysmal bone cyst: a review of 150 patients. J Clin Oncol 2005;23(27):6756–62.

65. Murphey MD, Andrews CL, Flemming DJ, et al. From the archives of the AFIP. Primary tumors of the spine: radiologic pathologic correlation. Radiographics 1996;16(5):1131–58.

66. Hudson TM, Hamlin DJ, Fitzsimmons JR. Magnetic resonance imaging of fluid levels in an aneurysmal bone cyst and in anticoagulated human blood. Skeletal Radiol 1985;13(4):267–70.

67. Bertram C, Madert J, Eggers C. Eosinophilic granuloma of the cervical spine. Spine 2002;27(13):1408–13.

68. Garg SS, Mehta SS, Dormans JPJ. Langerhans cell histiocytosis of the spine in children. Long-term follow-up. J Bone Joint Surg Am 2004;86-A(8):1740–50.

69. Gerber S, Ollivier L, Leclère J, et al. Imaging of sacral tumours. Skeletal Radiol 2008;37(4):277–89.

70. Yamaguchi TT, Watanabe-Ishiiwa HH, Suzuki SS, et al. Incipient chordoma: a report of two cases of early-stage chordoma arising from benign notochordal cell tumors. Mod Pathol 2005;18(7):1005–10.

71. Ulich TR, Mirra JM. Ecchordosis physaliphora vertebralis. Clin Orthop Relat Res 1982;(163):282–9.

72. Darby AJ, Cassar-Pullicino VN, McCall IW, Jaffray DC. Vertebral intra-osseous chordoma or giant notochordal rest? Skeletal Radiol 1999;28(6):342–6.

73. Mirra JM, Brien EW. Giant notochordal hamartoma of intraosseous origin: a newly reported benign entity to be distinguished from chordoma. Report of two cases. Skeletal Radiol 2001;30(12):698–709.

74. Yamaguchi T, Iwata J, Sugihara S, et al. Distinguishing benign notochordal cell tumors from vertebral chordoma. Skeletal Radiol 2008;37(4):291–9.

75. Nishiguchi T, Mochizuki K, Ohsawa M, et al. Differentiating benign notochordal cell tumors from chordomas: radiographic features on MRI, CT, and tomography. Am J Roentgenol 2011;196(3):644–50.

76. Terzi S, Mobarec S, Bandiera S, et al. Diagnosis and treatment of benign notochordal cell tumors of the spine: report of 3 cases and literature review. Spine 2012;37(21):E1356–60.

77. Farsad K, Kattapuram SV, Sacknoff R, et al. Sacral chordoma. Radiographics 2009;29(5):1525–30.

78. Smolders DD, Wang XX, Drevelengas AA, et al. Value of MRI in the diagnosis of non-clival, non-sacral chordoma. Skeletal Radiol 2003;32(6):343–50.

79. Boriani S, Bandiera S, Biagini R, et al. Chordoma of the mobile spine: fifty years of experience. Spine 2006;31(4):493–503.

80. Walcott BP, Nahed BV, Mohyeldin A, et al. Chordoma: current concepts, management, and future directions. Lancet Oncol 2012;13(2):e69–76.

81. Bjornsson JJ, Wold LEL, Ebersold MJM, Laws ERE. Chordoma of the mobile spine. A clinicopathologic analysis of 40 patients. Cancer 1993;71(3):735–40.

82. Wang Y, Xiao J, Wu Z, et al. Primary chordomas of the cervical spine: a consecutive series of 14 surgically managed cases. J Neurosurg Spine 2012;17(4):292–9.

83. Wippold FJF, Koeller KKK, Smirniotopoulos JGJ. Clinical and imaging features of cervical chordoma. Am J Roentgenol 1999;172(5):1423–6.

84. Sung MS, Lee GK, Kang HS, et al. Sacrococcygeal chordoma: MR imaging in 30 patients. Skeletal Radiol 2005;34(2):87–94.

85. Kwon JW, Chung HW, Cho EY, et al. MRI findings of giant cell tumors of the spine. Am J Roentgenol 2007;189(1):246–50.

86. Aoki JJ, Tanikawa HH, Ishii KK, et al. MR findings indicative of hemosiderin in giant-cell tumor of bone: frequency, cause, and diagnostic significance. Am J Roentgenol 1995;166(1):145–8.

87. Laredo JD, Quessar el A, Bossard P, Vuillemin-Bodaghi V. Vertebral tumors and pseudotumors. Radiol Clin North Am 2001;39(1):137–63, vi.

88. Murphey MD, Nomikos GC, Flemming DJ, et al. From the archives of AFIP. Imaging of giant cell tumor and giant cell reparative granuloma of bone: radiologic-pathologic correlation. Radiographics 2001;21(5):1283–309.

89. Sundaresan N, Rosen G, Boriani S. Primary malignant tumors of the spine. Orthop Clin North Am 2009;40(1):21–36.

90. Major NM, Helms CA, Richardson WJ. The 'mini brain': plasmacytoma in a vertebral body on MR imaging. Am J Roentgenol 2000;175(1):261–3.

91. Shah BKB, Saifuddin AA, Price GJG. Magnetic resonance imaging of spinal plasmacytoma. Clin Radiol 2000;55(6):439–45.

92. Mahnken AH, Wildberger JE, Gehbauer G, et al. Multidetector CT of the spine in multiple myeloma: comparison with MR imaging and radiography. Am J Roentgenol 2002;178(6):1429–36.

93. Lecouvet FE, Malghem J, Michaux L, et al. Vertebral compression fractures in multiple myeloma. Part II. Assessment of fracture risk with MR imaging of spinal bone marrow. Radiology 1997;204(1):201–5.

94. Murphey MD, Walker EA, Wilson AJ, et al. From the archives of the AFIP: imaging of primary chondrosarcoma: radiologic-pathologic correlation. Radiographics 2003;23(5):1245–78.

95. Boriani S, De Iure F, Bandiera S, et al. Chondrosarcoma of the mobile spine: report on 22 cases. Spine 2000;25(7):804–12.

96. Lloret I, Server A, Bjerkehagen B. Primary spinal chondrosarcoma: radiologic findings with pathologic correlation. Acta Radiol 2006;47(1):77–84.

97. Ilaslan HH, Sundaram MM, Unni KKK, Dekutoski MBM. Primary Ewing's sarcoma of the vertebral column. Skeletal Radiol 2004;33(9):506–13.

98. Mar WAW, Taljanovic MSM, Bagatell RR, et al. Update on imaging and treatment of Ewing sarcoma family tumors: what the radiologist needs to know. J Comput Assist Tomogr 2007;32(1):108–18.

99. Ilaslan HH, Sundaram MM, Unni KKK, Shives TCT. Primary vertebral osteosarcoma: imaging findings. Radiology 2004;230(3):697–702.

CHAPTER 4

NON-TUMOURAL SPINAL CORD LESIONS

Farah Alobeidi • Majda M. Thurnher • H. Rolf Jäger

INFLAMMATORY DISEASE

Multiple Sclerosis

Multiple sclerosis (MS) is a progressive neurodegenerative disorder characterised by multiple inflammatory demyelinating foci called 'plaques'. The spinal cord is commonly involved with changes on autopsy in up to 98% of the cases. One-third of MS patients will have isolated spinal cord involvement. Spinal cord abnormalities in MS include focal lesions, diffuse involvement, axonal loss and spinal cord atrophy. Focal MS lesions appear as oval- or wedge-shaped T_2 hyperintensities located preferentially in the lateral and posterior parts of the spinal cord, which may or may not be swollen. Lesion enhancement is seen less frequently than in the brain, and is commonly subtle (Fig. 4-1). Ring-like or intense nodular enhancement may also occur.

Diffuse signal intensity abnormalities extending over multiple vertebral segments resembling transverse myelitis are seen in primary and secondary progressive MS. Spinal cord atrophy is associated with clinical disability, and is more common in the upper part of the spinal cord.

Tumefactive MS lesions can sometimes present a diagnostic challenge with a clinical presentation and imaging features mimicking tumours. Magnetic resonance imaging (MRI) appearances are classically of large (greater than 2 cm) circumscribed lesions with little mass effect or oedema. They are typically found in the supratentorial white matter but can also involve grey matter and the spinal cord (Fig. 4-2). Approximately half of tumefactive lesions enhance with a typical open ring pattern, with the incomplete portion of the ring on the grey matter side of the lesion (Fig. 4-2). Corticosteroid therapy leads to a dramatic reduction in the size of the lesions.

Acute Disseminated Encephalomyelitis

Acute disseminated encephalomyelitis (ADEM) is an inflammatory demyelinating cental nervous system (CNS) disease of the brain and spinal cord, with a distinct tendency to a perivenous localisation of pathological changes. ADEM develops mostly one or two weeks following a viral disease or prior vaccinations. Cerebrospinal fluid (CSF) analysis shows a high protein level. A high serum titre of IgG specific for myelin oligodendrocyte glycoprotein (MOG) has been described in almost one-half of the studied cases of ADEM.[1]

The spinal cord is involved in 30–40% of the cases. On MR imaging, non-enhancing hyperintense lesions are seen in the spinal cord on long TR sequences (Fig. 4-3). Skip lesions, as well as long segment hyperintensity, may be detected. Complete resolution of abnormalities will usually be seen on follow-up images.

Acute Transverse Myelitis

Acute transverse myelitis (ATM) is an aetiologically heterogeneous syndrome with acute or subacute onset, manifesting as weakness, sensory loss and autonomic dysfunction. It is associated with infectious or systemic autoimmune diseases, but in the majority of cases the aetiology remains unknown (idiopathic). In 2002 diagnostic criteria for idiopathic and disease-associated ATM were proposed by the Transverse Myelitis Consortium Working Group.[2]

The outcome of ATM ranges from full recovery to complete inability to walk or even death from respiratory failure. On MR imaging, intramedullary T_2 high signal intensity with cord swelling will be seen. Enhancement may be present. In comparison with spinal cord involvement in MS where focal lesion do not take more than half of the cross-sectional area of the cord, lesions in TM tend to involve more than two-thirds of the cross-sectional area of the cord (Fig. 4-4).

Depending on the length of the signal abnormality, TM can be divided into longitudinally extensive TM (LETM) when signal abnormalities extend more than two segments and acute partial TM (APTM) when signal abnormalities extend less than two vertebral segments.

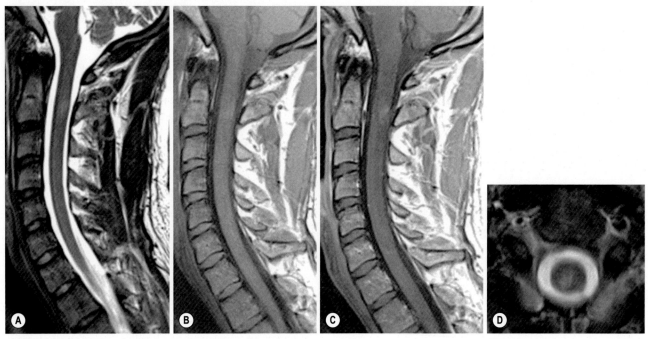

FIGURE 4-1 ≡ **Multiple sclerosis in a 30-year-old female patient.** (A) Sagittal T_2 demonstrates an ill-defined hyperintense lesion in the spinal cord at the level of C2. The lesion is isointense on T_1 (B) and shows subtle enhancement on post-contrast T_1 (C). (D) Axial T_2 shows dorsal location of the demyelinating plaque.

Neuromyelitis Optica

Neuromyelitis optica (NMO) is a severe inflammatory disorder that predominantly affects the optic nerves and the spinal cord. It has a relapsing course in 80% of the cases and females are more commonly affected (9:1). The discovery of aquaporin-4 antibodies in 2004 has substantially changed our understanding of the disease, which was for many years debated and considered as an MS subtype.[3] Antibodies to aquaporin-4 (AQP4-Ab or NMO-IgG) are sensitive and highly specific serum markers of NMO, and will be positive in 60–90% of NMO patients. Patients with NMO present either with optic neuritis (unilateral or bilateral) or with LETM and spinal symptoms.

In optic neuritis MRI shows hyperintensity of the optic nerves with enhancement. Spinal cord involvement manifests itself as intramedullary T_2 hyperintense signal often extending more than three vertebral segments (LETM) with cavitations and patchy enhancement. On follow-up magnetic resonance (MR) defects, atrophy and central cavities, predominately located in the area of the posterior fascicle, have been described.[4] In some cases MRI findings may resemble spinal cord ischaemia with bilateral ventral hyperintensities.[4] Contrary to the common belief that brain lesions are not present in NMO, recent studies reported brain abnormalities in up to 40–60% of NMO patients. Periventricular signal intensity abnormalities (around the third and fourth ventricle, and in the periaqueductal region) can be detected on MRI, corresponding to brain areas with the highest aquaporin concentrations. Extensive lesions in the cerebral hemispheres have also been described.[5] Enhancement on brain MRI is

not common (13–36%), with 'cloud-like enhancement', which appears as multiple patches of enhancing lesions being the most common type.[6]

NMO has been associated with other autoimmune diseases, including hypothyroidism, Sjögren's syndrome (SS), systemic lupus erythematosus (SLE), pernicious anaemia, ulcerative colitis, primary sclerosing cholangitis, rheumatoid arthritis, mixed connective tissue disorders and idiopathic thrombocytopenic purpura.

Systemic Lupus Erythematosus

Systemic lupus erythematosus (SLE) is a relapsing and remitting, chronic, multisystem autoimmune disease. Although the frequency of neuropsychiatric lupus has been reported as high as 95%, SLE-related myelitis is rare, with prevalence varying between 1 and 2%. Involvement of the spinal cord in SLE usually occurs during a time of acute exacerbation and is occasionally the first manifestation of SLE in an undiagnosed patient.

SLE myelitis manifests mostly as transverse myelopathy. The pathophysiological mechanism of TM in SLE is uncertain, although vasculitis and arterial thrombosis resulting in ischaemic cord necrosis have been suggested. Studies have suggested a higher incidence of antiphospholipid and NMO-IgG antibodies in those with SLE myelitis than in the general SLE population and this has contributed to our understanding of the disease process.[7]

The mid-thoracic cord is most commonly affected, resulting in a sensory level and frequently in paraplegia, which may be complete. Cervical myelopathy and cauda equina involvement, on the other hand, often cause only partial motor and sensory loss. MRI demonstrates T_2

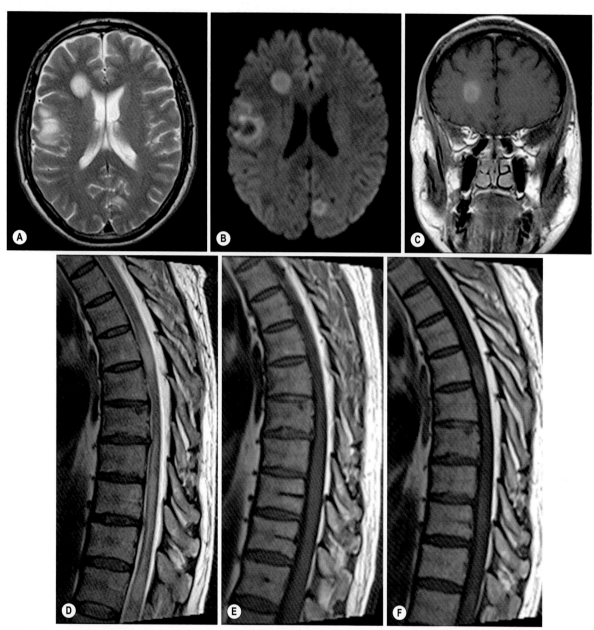

FIGURE 4-2 ■ Tumefactive MS. (A) Axial T_2 demonstrating multiple hyperintense lesions within the right frontal and left occipital lobes. The lesions are relatively well defined with little mass effect. Other lesions were also present (not shown). (B) DWI shows a rim of restricted diffusion in the larger lesion; the ring is incomplete laterally, which is a typical finding in tumefactive MS lesions. (C) Coronal post-contrast T_1 demonstrating enhancement of the right frontal lobe lesion. (D) Sagittal T_2 of the thoracic spine demonstrating multiple T_2 hyperintense lesions, the caudal of which extends over several segments. The lesions are not clearly seen on (E) sagittal T_1, but demonstrate ring-like enhancement post-contrast administration on (F) sagittal T_1 post contrast.

hyperintensity and oedema, frequently with spinal cord expansion. Lesions may demonstrate patchy enhancement during the acute phase (Fig. 4-5). Improvement or resolution of these findings correlates with clinical improvement. Indeed, some patients may have a normal MRI if they have already received treatment.

Sarcoidosis

Sarcoidosis is a systemic condition of unknown aetiology characterised histologically by non-caseating granulomatosis. Although CNS sarcoidosis is found in approximately 25% of cases on post-mortem examination, symptomatic involvement in life is uncommon. Clinical presentation depends on the site of involvement and is often non-specific.

Spinal involvement may be osseous, discal, meningeal or involve the cord itself. The most common spinal cord manifestation is leptomeningeal enhancement. This is best seen on sagittal contrast-enhanced T_1 images as thin linear or nodular enhancement, which frequently extends along the surface of the nerve roots. Dural

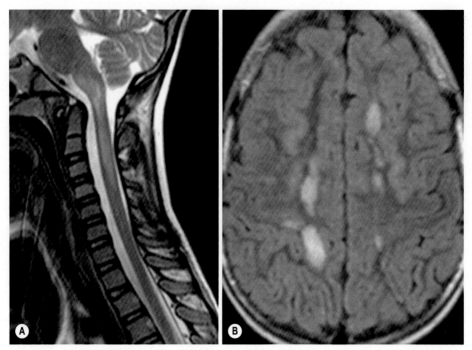

FIGURE 4-3 ■ **Acute disseminated encephalomyelitis (ADEM) with brain and spinal cord involvement in a child with acute onset of symptoms following viral infection.** (A) Sagittal T_2 of the cervical spine shows homogeneous high-signal-intensity abnormality in the cervical spinal cord and medulla oblongata. On post-contrast T_1 no enhancement is observed (not shown). (B) On an axial FLAIR MR image of the brain, multiple hyperintense white matter lesions are detected.

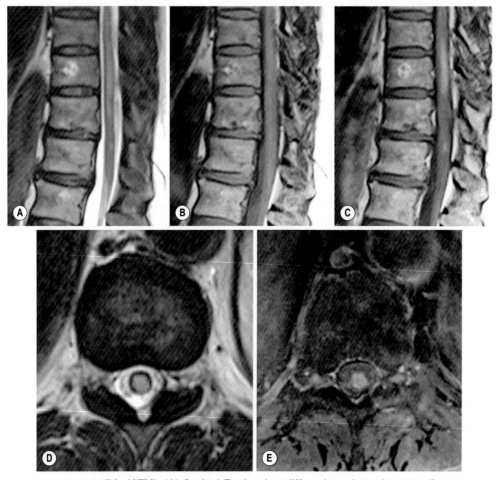

FIGURE 4-4 ■ **Acute transverse myelitis (ATM).** (A) Sagittal T_2 showing diffuse hyperintensity extending over several segments. Sagittal T_1 pre four (B) and post four (C) contrast showing enhancement of the lesion. Axial T_2 (D) and axial post-contrast T_1 (E) demonstrate that the lesion occupies more than two-thirds of the spinal cord cross-section.

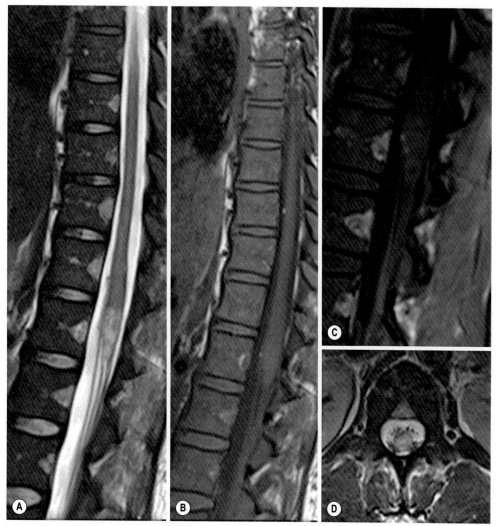

FIGURE 4-5 ■ **Systemic lupus erythematosus.** (A) Sagittal T_2 and (B) sagittal T_1 of the thoracolumbar spine demonstrating a lesion within the conus medullaris. A smaller, similar-appearing lesion was present in the same patient in the cervical spine (not shown). (C) Magnified post-contrast sagittal T_1 sagittal show faint enhancement of the lesion. (D) On axial T_2 the lesion occupies most of the transverse section of the conus medullaris.

involvement is more nodular in appearance, often with enhancing dural-based mass-like lesions that may mimic meningiomas.

Intramedullary spinal lesions are uncommon and frequently associated with severe neurological deficit. MRI demonstrates an enhancing mass that is hyperintense on T_2 sequences with associated fusiform enlargement of the spinal cord. These findings are, however, non-specific and can mimic intramedullary tumours, TM, MS and fungal infections. When the cauda equina is involved there is enhancement and clumping of the nerve roots.

The diagnosis of CNS sarcoidosis can represent a challenge on spinal cord imaging alone and is supported by the presence of typical appearances of brain sarcoidosis, such as involvement of the hypothalamic–pituitary axis, leptomeningeal enhancement or dural masses, as well as other diagnostic tests, such as elevated serum ACE levels.

DEMYELINATING POLYNEUROPATHIES

Although not strictly diseases of the spinal cord, demyelinating polyneuropathies merit a brief mention here as they can affect the cauda equina and other intradural nerves, leading to abnormal findings on an MRI of the spine.

Guillain–Barré Syndrome

Guillain–Barré is an acute immune-mediated polyneuropathy. Affected individuals have a typical areflexia and ascending paralysis type of symmetrical weakness, with or without sensory loss, that starts in the feet and hands and progressively moves up the limbs to the trunk over a few days. The trigger is frequently a viral illness with the production of antibodies that cross-react with myelin in the peripheral nervous system.[8] Approximately 80%

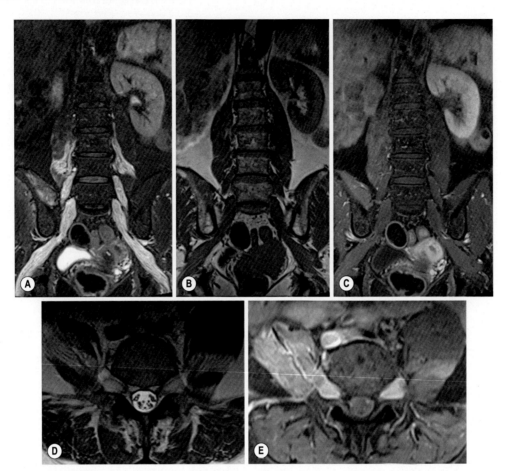

FIGURE 4-6 ■ **Chronic inflammatory demyelinating polyneuropathy (CIDP).** Coronal (A) fat-suppressed (FS) T_2 demonstrating grossly enlarged T_2 hyperintense nerves. (B) Pre-contrast T_1 and (C) FS post-contrast T_1 show diffusion enhancement of the nerves. Note that there is asymmetry of the psoas and pelvic muscles with atrophy, T_2 hyperintensity and enhancement typical for acute denervation. (D) Axial T_2 at level of L4 and (E) axial post-contrast FS T_1 confirm T_2 hyperintensity and enhancement of both the intradural and extradural nerves as well as the asymmetry and enhancement of the psoas muscles.

make complete or near-complete recovery over a few weeks from onset, with approximately 10% developing persistent symptoms that may have a relapsing and remitting course. In approximately 10% of cases, it can be life threatening if the respiratory muscles are affected.

Diagnosis is usually clinical and supplemented by nerve conduction studies and CSF examination. MRI demonstrates nerve thickening and enhancement, which is non-specific and is seen in other inflammatory disorders but is a useful diagnostic adjunct.

Chronic Inflammatory Demyelinating Polyneuropathy (CIDP)

This is an immune-mediated chronically progressive or relapsing symmetric sensorimotor disorder. It can be considered the chronic equivalent of acute inflammatory demyelinating polyneuropathy, the most common form of Guillain–Barré syndrome. In contrast to Guillain–Barré syndrome, CIDP has an insidious onset and evolves in either a slowly progressive or a relapsing manner. Preceding infection is infrequent. As with

Guillain–Barré syndrome, the mainstay of treatment is immunosuppressive or immunomodulatory intervention. MRI findings are similar, with enhancing thickened nerve roots. Acute and subacute muscle denervation is demonstrated by hyperintensity within the affected muscle on fluid-sensitive sequences, such as T_2-weighted or STIR images. In chronic denervation, muscle atrophy and fatty infiltration demonstrate high signal changes on T_1-weighted sequences in association with volume loss. CIDP may therefore show both these changes depending on the stage of imaging (Fig. 4-6).

VASCULAR DISEASES

Spinal Dural Arteriovenous Fistula (SDAVF)

Over 80% of spinal arteriovenous malformations represent SDAVFs located in the spinal dural mater, usually close to a root sleeve.[9] Such fistulae are most commonly located in the thoracolumbar region but can occur at any

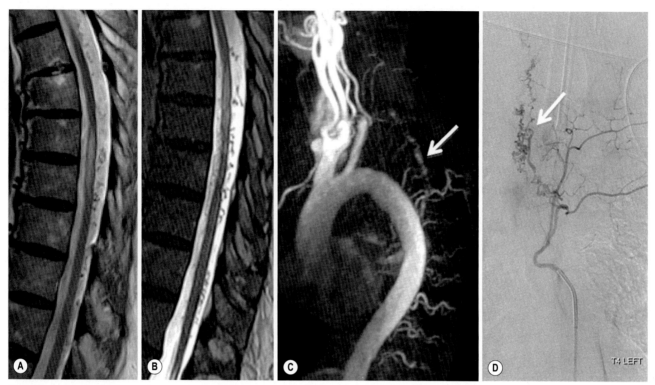

FIGURE 4-7 ■ **Spinal dural arteriovenous fistula (SDAVF).** (A) Sagittal T_2 demonstrating intrinsic T_2 cord hyperintensity in keeping with spinal cord oedema. Serpiginous flow voids of the dilated perimedullary veins are more prominent on the dorsal surface and appear more conspicuous on (B) the CISS sequence. (C) Sagittal reconstruction of TWIST sequence at the level of the thoracic aorta suggests presence of a fistula in the upper thoracic cord (arrow). A SDAVF was confirmed by DSA (D) following selective catheterisation of left supreme intercostal trunk which demonstrated the fistulous point (arrow).

level, though in the cervical spine only around the foramen magnum except in extremely rare cases. The fistula is usually supplied by one or two branches of a nearby radiculomeningeal artery and shunts often via a single vein into intradural radicular veins. The increase in spinal venous pressure results in slow venous drainage and stagnation because radicular veins and intramedullary veins share a common venous outflow. This results in the clinical findings of progressive myelopathy. SDAVFs are more common in middle-aged to elderly men and the typical presentation is of a slowly progressive gait disturbance, difficulty climbing stairs and paraesthesia. Bowel and bladder incontinence, erectile dysfunction and urinary retention are often seen late in the course of the disease but may be the presenting feature.

Diagnosis is often made by radiologists, based on typical MRI imaging features that guide definitive diagnosis by spinal DSA. T_2 sequences show an ill-defined central intramedullary hyperintensity extending over multiple levels with associated cord expansion. There may be a hypointense rim, most likely due to deoxygenated blood within dilated capillary vessels surrounding the congested oedema.[10] Engorged perimedullary veins can be seen as flow voids, which are more pronounced on the dorsal surface compared to the ventral surface. Although these are readily depicted on standard T_2 sequences, they become much more conspicuous on

heavily T_2-weighted sequences (constructive interference in steady state (CISS), fast imaging employing steady-state acquisition (FIESTA) or 3D turbo spin-echo (3D TSE)) (Fig. 4-7). There may be diffuse post-contrast enhancement of the spinal cord, reflecting breakdown of the blood–brain barrier. The coiled perimedullary veins are easily depicted following contrast enhancement. It should be noted that normal pial veins can be prominent at the level of the lumbar enlargement of the spinal cord and that the distribution of abnormally enlarged veins is a poor guide to the location of a dural fistula. The site of the fistula can, however, be sometimes shown by dynamic contrast-enhanced magnetic resonance angiography (MRA). Multiplanar reformats of 4D dynamic MRA sequences, such as time-resolved angiography with interleaved stochastic trajectories (TWIST), can show non-invasively the site of the SDAVF in cases where the diagnosis is uncertain and can guide digital subtraction angiography (DSA), helping to avoid unnecessary superselective injections of all possible arterial feeders (Fig. 4-7).[11]

These lesions are an absolute indication for DSA. When searching for a dural fistula, imaging should be slow, say one frame rate every 2 s due to delayed venous return. A large number of arteries may have to be injected before the lesion is found. The study should not be regarded as negative unless: (A) all the spinal arteries from the foramen magnum to the coccyx have been opacified adequately, or (B) the veins thought to be abnormal have been opacified and shown to drain normally.[12] If a lesion is found, adjacent levels should also be injected and the major radiculomedullary arteries supplying the region must be identified.

Treatment aims to stop disease progression, with prognosis dependent on the symptoms and stage of disease pre-treatment. Embolisation of arteries supplying a dural fistula may be feasible, provided the vessel to be embolised can also be shown *not* to supply the spinal cord. The aim of treatment is to exclude the shunting zone (i.e. the most distal part of the artery together with the most proximal part of the draining vein).[13] Of course this is not always possible and a more proximal occlusion will lead to a transient improvement of symptoms, although fistula recurrence is high in these cases. Early surgical intervention should be considered for incomplete embolisations, as delay of secondary intervention is associated with a poor outcome.[14]

Spinal Arteriovenous Malformations (SAVMs)

In contrast to SDAVFs, spinal arteriovenous malformations (AVMs) are fed by spinal arteries, either radicullomedullary and/or radicullopial, located in an intra- or perimedullary location, respectively. There are two distinct subtypes: (A) glomerular AVMs (also known as plexiform or nidus type), the most common, contain a cluster or nidus of abnormal vessels between the feeding artery and draining vein and (B) fistulous AVMs (also known as AVM of the perimedullary fistula type or intradural AV fistula) which are direct AV shunts commonly located superficially on the cord.[15] Drainage is via spinal cord veins or perimedullary veins. In contrast to SDAVFs, these lesions are more prone to haemorrhage, a useful discriminating feature on MRI. Depending on the AVM location, haemorrhage may be intramedullary or subarachnoid. Lesions can also cause symptoms via venous congestion in a pathophysiology mechanism similar to SDAVF.

The dilated intra- and/or perimedullary veins are demonstrated on MRI as serpiginous flow voids on T_2 sequences, which enhance post-contrast administration. If there is venous congestion, oedema is present, seen as ill-defined intramedullary T_2 hyperintensity with cord expansion. If haemorrhage is present, various intramedullary signal intensities are seen, depending on the age of the blood. A subarachnoid haemorrhage may be present. There may also be an intranidal aneurysm (Fig. 4-8).

Embolisation of AVMs can sometimes be therapeutic but frequently it is palliative or 'targeted' to eliminate false aneurysms or to reduce hypertension or as a precursor to surgical treatment.

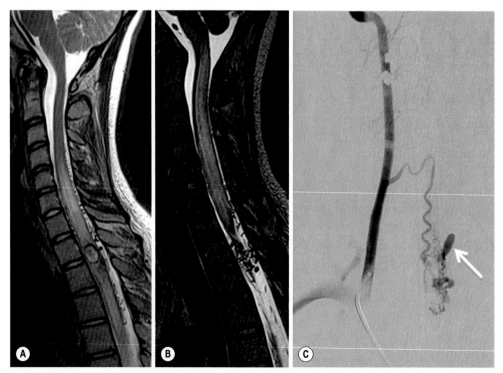

FIGURE 4-8 ■ **Spinal arteriovenous malformation (SAVM).** (A) Sagittal T_2 MRI demonstrating an intramedullary lesion at $T_{1/2}$ with a hypointense rim in keeping with haemosiderosis. Note the cord expansion and associated cord oedema. Note also the serpiginous flow voids, which are more prominent on the dorsal surface of the cord. These are much more conspicuous on heavily weighted T_2 sequences such as (B) CISS sequence, right parasagittal slice. (C) Selective catheterisation of the right vertebral artery on DSA confirms the presence of an arteriovenous malformation. Note the intranidal aneurysm (arrow).

TABLE 4-1   **Summary of Spinal Vascular Malformations and Fistulas**

Type	Angio-architecture	Age (years)	Typical Clinical Presentation	Haemorrhage	Notes
Dural	Fistula	40–70	Progressive myelopathy	Rare	Male predominance, rarely cervical
Perimedullary (type I) (micro)	Fistula	30–70	Progressive myelopathy	Rare	Clinical and MR findings mimic SDAVF
Perimedullary (type II) (micro)	Fistula	20–40	Acute neurological deficit	Common	Commonly at conus
Perimedullary (type III) (macro)	Fistula	2–30	Acute neurological deficit	Common	Associated with Oslu–Weber–Rendu
Intramedullary	Nidus	10–40	Acute neurological deficit	Common	Flow-related aneurysms
Extradural	Fistula	Any	Asymptomatic to progressive myelopathy	Rare	Symptoms due to venous drainage pattern
Complex	Fistula	5–20	Acute or progressive neurological deficits	Common	Partial treatment often best pattern

A summary of SDAVFs and spinal AVMs, together with other types of vascular malformations and fistulas, is shown in Table 4-1.[16]

Spinal Cord Cavernous Malformation (SCCM)

Cavernous malformations (also known as cavernomas, cavernous angiomas and cavernous haemangiomas) are vascular malformations composed of sinusoidal-type vessels in immediate apposition to each other without any normal intervening parenchyma. In contrast to the brain where they are relatively common, SCCMs are more rare. They can be extradural, intradural-extramedullary or most commonly, intramedullary. Four clinical presentation subtypes have been described:[17] (A) discrete episodes of neurological deterioration separated by variable time intervals (hours or days) during which various degrees of recovery are made; (B) slowly progressive myelopathy; (C) acute neurological deficit with rapid decline; and (D) acute neurological deficit with gradual decline over weeks or months. Small repeated haemorrhages have been suggested as the underlying pathophysiological mechanism for episodes of repeated acute neurological deficit.

MRI appearances are characteristic with heterogeneous lesions on both T_1- and T_2-weighted sequences displaying typical 'popcorn' appearances, due to blood products of different ages. Due to haemosiderin staining, there is a T_2 low-intensity rim and hypointense 'blooming' on gradient-echo sequences. There may be minimal contrast enhancement, cord expansion or oedema (Fig. 4-9).

Symptomatic SCCM should be surgically removed at an early stage to avoid recurrence or rebleeding.[17]

Spinal Cord Infarction

In contrast to its cranial counterpart, spinal cord infarction is rare due to its rich anastomotic blood supply.

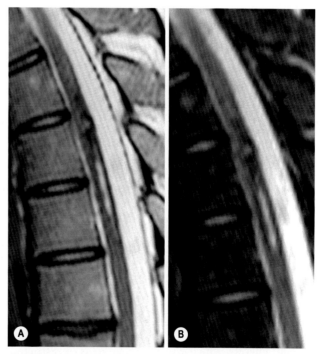

FIGURE 4-9 ■ **Spinal cord cavernous malformation (SCCM).** (A) Sagittal T_2 and (B) with fat suppression demonstrating intramedullary lesion with heterogeneous signal intensity and T_2 hypointense rim in keeping with blood products. Note the associated intrinsic cord T_2 hyperintensity, which extends for several segments above and below the lesion.

Complication following aortic aneurysm repair and aortic dissection are the most common causes of spinal cord infarction, although frequently no definite case is identified. Clinical presentation is acute, evolving over minutes, in contrast to other myelopathies and spinal cord lesions. The neurological deficit is frequently bilateral and accompanied by pain, with symptoms dependent on the level of involvement. Spinal cord infarcts are more often located in the thoracolumbar cord than the cervical cord and are frequently located

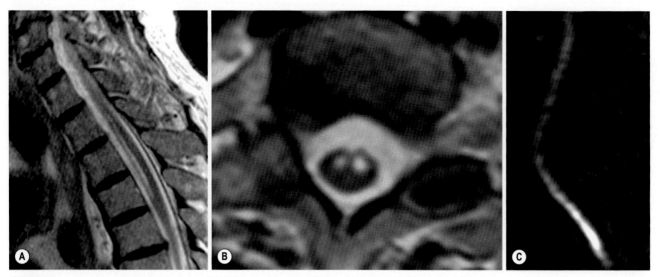

FIGURE 4-10 ■ **Acute spinal cord ischaemia with acute onset of symptoms in a male patient following aortic repair.** (A) On sagittal T_2 of the cervicothoracic spine linear hyperintensity is shown in the ventral part of the spinal cord extending over three vertebral segments. (B) Axial T_2 demonstrates 'snake's eyes' appearance, indicating involvement of the ventral grey matter of the spinal cord. (C) Sagittal trace DWI demonstrates high signal consistent with restricted diffusion.

in the central and anterior territories of the anterior spinal artery. This results in a classical sensory pattern loss of superficial pain and temperature discrimination, with relative preservation of light touch, vibration and position sense. Weakness and sensory loss for all techniques are found at the segmental levels of the spinal cord infarct.

In acute cases, MRI demonstrates high T_2 signal intensity in the central aspect of the cord; this may result in an 'owl's eyes' or 'snake's eyes' appearance on axial imaging through the lesion due to involvement on the anterior part of the grey matter. There will be some enhancement on post-contrast imaging due to breakdown of the blood–brain barrier. Diffusion-weighted imaging (DWI) is particularly sensitive to acute ischaemic change and should be performed in suspected cases of acute infarcts, which will appear as areas of restricted diffusion (Fig. 4-10).

Spinal Cord Vasculitis

Vasculitis of the spinal cord can be primary or idiopathic, known as primary angitis of the CNS, or secondary to a wide range of immune-mediated and inflammatory conditions such as SLE, Sjögren's and Behçet's disease to name a few.

MRI demonstrates multiple T_2 hyperintense focal intramedullary lesions. On axial images, these are frequently located in the dorsal and lateral aspects of the cord, resembling MS plaques. In the acute phase the lesions enhance following contrast administration and similar lesions can also be shown in the brain (Fig. 4-11). Follow-up MRI studies will show regression of the enhancement of some/all of the lesions.

Imaging findings are non-specific, with a wide differential diagnosis including MS, ADEM, sarcoidosis, infections and metastases, which have been discussed elsewhere in this and other chapters. A diagnosis of spinal vasculitis should only be made after clinical correlation, a review of the brain imaging and results of other diagnostic tests.

SPINAL CORD INFECTION

Spinal cord infection can be bacterial, viral, fungal or parasitic in origin.

Bacterial spinal cord abscess is a rare entity, with epidural abscess being far more common. In most described cases of *Staphylococcus aureus* abscesses, meningitis and epidural abscess were simultaneously present. Bacterial spinal cord abscesses have been described in intravenous drug abusers, in the setting of an intracardiac right-to-left shunt, following lumbar puncture, and also in otherwise healthy individuals. On MRI, bacterial intramedullary abscesses will have ring-like or peripheral enhancement, high-signal-intensity centre and marked spinal cord oedema.

Tuberculous spinal cord abscess is a rare form of spinal tuberculosis, compared to extradural collections in tuberculous spondylodiscitis. The lesions exhibit low signal intensity on T_1 and high signal on T_2 with peripheral enhancement of the capsule. In cases of tuberculous myelitis T_2 hyperintensity in the spinal cord with or without enhancement will be observed (Fig. 4-12). Intramedullary tuberculoma is rare and the thoracic cord is the most common location. The MRI appearance is characterised by hypointense ring enhancement, with or without

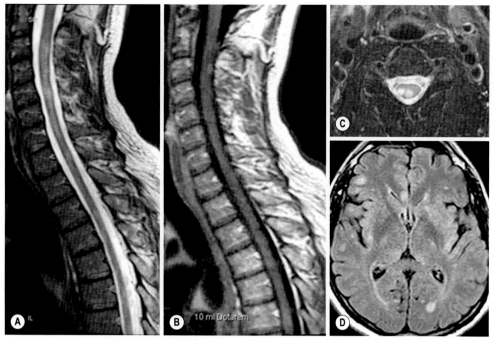

FIGURE 4-11 ■ **Vasculitis with brain and spinal cord involvement.** (A) The sagittal STIR images show multiple focal hyperintense lesions. (B) Only one of these lesions (at the level of C3) shows a subtle enhancement on post-contrast T_1. (C) Axial fat-suppressed T_2 confirms that the lesions are located in the dorsal and lateral parts of the spinal cord, resembling MS lesions. (D) Multiple focal lesions are seen on an axial FLAIR image of the brain.

central hyperintensity on T_2 images and hypo- to isointense rings on T_1 images.

Viral myelitis seen in immunocompromised individuals is mostly due to cytomegalovirus (CMV) infection, and is a common complication after solid organ transplantations. Imaging findings are non-specific with intramedullary T_2 hyperintensity (Fig. 4-13). Varicellazoster virus (VZV) may also cause myelitis with similar imaging appearances and can occur in immunocompetent as well as immunocompromised individuals.

Fungal spinal cord infections are due to *Aspergillus* or *Candida* species and are mostly seen in immunocompromised patients.

Parasitic myelitis is rare, and has been described in toxoplasmosis and cysticercosis. Patients with toxoplasmic myelitis almost always have cerebral involvement. On MRI, enhancing intramedullary lesions with extensive cord oedema will be seen. Although spinal cord toxoplasmosis is uncommon, in AIDS patients presenting with evolving myelopathy and enhancing lesions in brain and/or spinal cord toxoplasmic myelitis should be considered.

In intramedullary cysticercosis the appearance on MRI depends on the stage. In the early vesicular stage there is a well-defined T_2 hyperintense cyst in the spinal cord. On T_1 the cyst will have low signal intensity with high-signal-intensity scolex. In a later stage (colloidal stage) the thickened cyst capsule shows high signal on T_1 and low signal on T_2. The cyst content appears hyperintense on T_1 and scolex becomes invisible. Peripheral enhancement is seen in cyst degeneration.

DEVELOPMENTAL AND CYST-LIKE LESIONS

The commonest congenital malformation found in adults involves the caudal part of the neural tube. A useful descriptive term is lipomyelomeningodysplasia, which emphasises the various elements. Other conditions result in a dorsal dermal sinus that runs from a skin dimple to the spinal canal, some terminating in intraspinal dermoids or epidermoids. The neuroenteric canal or adhesion may persist, or form at other levels such as the upper cervical region, resulting in neuroenteric cysts along the connection between the foregut and spinal canal; a persistent cutaneous communication results in a dorsal enteric fistula. Aberrant neuro-endodermal adhesions are probably also the origin of diastematomyelia. Finally, excessive retrogressive differentiation can lead to various degrees of sacral and sacrolumbar dysgenesis, often referred to as the caudal regression syndromes.

Intramedullary Lipoma

This consists of a mass of adipose tissue located mainly between the posterior columns of the spinal cord. A tongue-like extension along the central canal is often found, in keeping with its embryogenesis. The overlying dura mater is usually intact and the lipoma entirely intradural; however, there may be a dural defect to which spinal cord and lipoma become adherent. Such

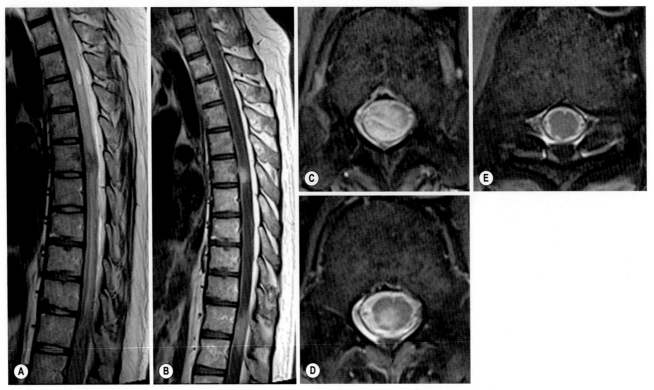

FIGURE 4-12 ■ **Spinal TB in male recently moved from India.** (A) Sagittal T_2 of the thoracic spine demonstrating multiple intramedullary lesions, of different signal intensities and associated widespread T_2 hyperintensity. These findings are in keeping with TB granulomata and associated spinal cord oedema. The most inferior lesion on this image has a T_2 hypointense rim suggestive of haemorrhage. (B) Following contrast enhancement, some of the lesions enhance. Note also the extensive leptomeningeal enhancement, particularly along the ventral aspect. There is also patchy intramedullary enhancement at the cervicothoracic junction. (C–E) A series of axial contrast-enhanced T_1 through the lower thoracic cord demonstrate cord expansion and enhancement of the intramedullary lesion as well as of the surrounding leptomeninges and CSF space, which appears bright, mimicking a T_2 sequence.

lesions occur most often near the thoracocervical or craniovertebral junction. CT and MRI demonstrate the fatty nature of the tumour. They may be associated with other conditions such as diastomatomyelia (Fig. 4-14). Non-fatty elements may also be present, resulting in a heterogeneous appearance.

Lipomyelomeningodysplasias

These represent a spectrum of abnormalities ranging from an abnormally low location of the conus medullaris with minimal or even absent lipoma, to massive lipomatous formations involving all elements of the spinal and adjacent subcutaneous tissues. The abnormality may not be apparent clinically, hence the term occult spinal dysraphism. Unlike myelocele, Chiari malformation is present in only 6%. Patients frequently present in adult life, sometimes only with back pain and minimal neurological signs.

MR is the optimal investigation, although ultrasound (US) has been advocated in children. MR demonstrates all aspects of the abnormalities including the origin of nerve roots and associated lesions such as cysts in the spinal cord. In over 80%, the spinal cord terminates at or below the level of the third lumbar vertebra, and is usually tethered to the dorsal aspect of the dura, where it fuses with the fatty tumour. Nerve roots issuing from an apparently thickened filum terminale indicate that it contains significant nervous tissue and therefore should not be divided surgically.

Diastematomyelia

The spinal cord is split into two usually unequal hemicords, each with a central canal and anterior spinal artery, but giving rise to only ipsilateral spinal roots. Any level can be involved, including the filum terminale and medulla oblongata, but most are thoracic.[18] The cleavage usually extends over several segments and only rarely do the hemicords not reunite caudally. The hemicords are enclosed in a common dural tube in 50% of cases, usually in the cervical region, but in the remainder each is enclosed in its own dural tube, with a bony or cartillagenous spur arising from malformed lamina often lying between them. Abnormal traction may be exerted by such a spur at the point of reunion of the hemicords. Clinical abnormalities are often absent, but in some symptomatic cases progression apparently was halted by excision of tethering spurs. MRI shows the abnormality well (Fig. 4-14).

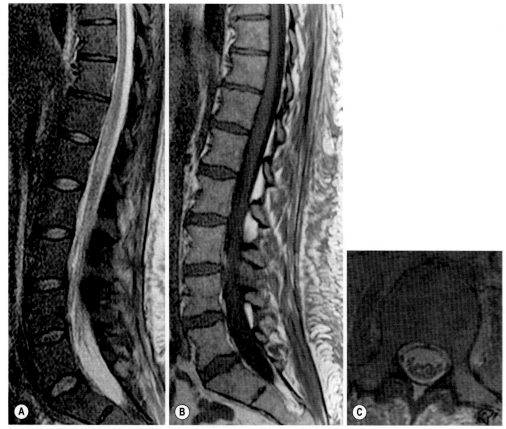

FIGURE 4-13 ■ **Cytomegalovirus (CMV) myelitis in an immunocompromised patient after heart transplantation.** (A) On sagittal STIR images subtle high signal intensity is detected in the conus medullaris. (B) On sagittal post-contrast T_1 images only subtle enhancement and clumping of cauda equina was detected on (C) axial T_2. In the CSF analysis PCR was positive for CMV.

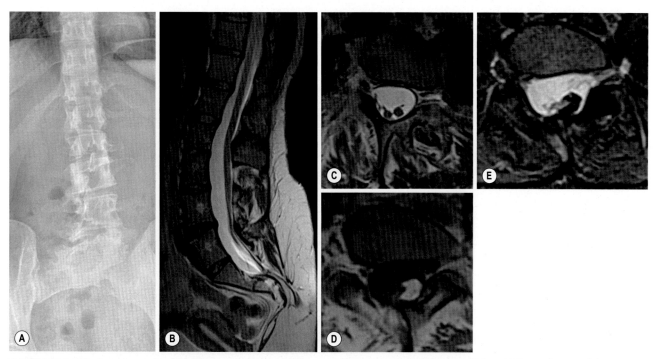

FIGURE 4-14 ■ **Diastematomyelia.** (A) AP thoracolumbar radiograph demonstrating deformity of L4 and L5 vertebrae and the sacrum with absence of the coccyx. There is a mild lumbar scoliosis concave to the right. (B) Sagittal T_1 of the lumbar spine demonstrating an ill-defined low-lying conus at the L4–L5 level. The nerve roots are tethered caudally and herniate through a bony defect in the posterior elements. There is agenesis of the lower sacrum and the coccyx. (C) Axial T_2 through the lower thoracic spine clearly demonstrates the split cord. (D) Axial T_1 through the lower dural sac demonstrates an intradural extramedullary left-sided high-signal-intensity lesion. This suppresses on (E) fat-suppressed axial T_2 at the same level. The appearances are in keeping with a lipoma.

Neuroenteric and Other Developmental Cysts

Intraspinal neuroenteric cysts are intradural, usually unilocular cysts lined by gastrointestinal or bronchial epithelium that occur in either the cervical (often near the craniovertebral junction) or lower thoracic regions.[19]

They compress the spinal cord (usually the anterior aspect) and may invaginate into its substance; occasionally the spinal cord is split into two halves as in diastematomyelia. Plain radiography may show focal expansion of the spinal canal, and thoracic lesions in particular may be associated with butterfly or hemivertebrae (Fig. 4-15). On MRI the cyst contents may yield a slightly higher

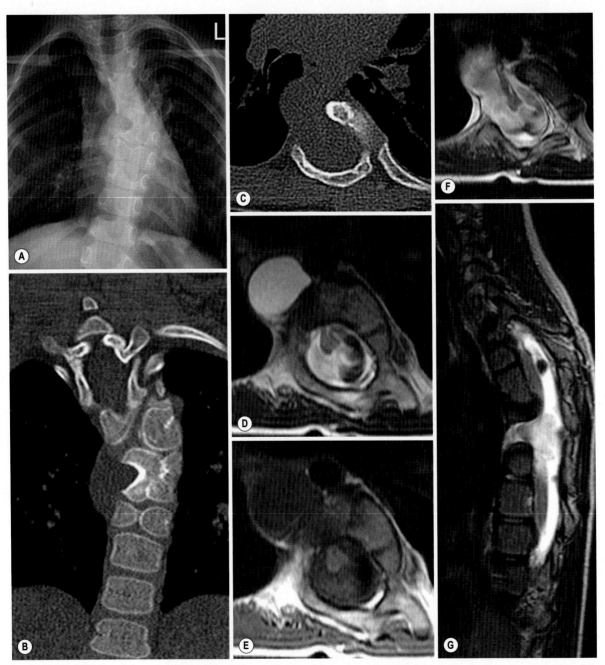

FIGURE 4-15 ■ **Neuroenteric cyst.** (A) Chest radiograph and (B) coronal multiplanar reformat of CT thorax in same patient. There is a complex segmentation anomaly within the mid-thoracic region associated with kyphoscoliosis, consisting of congenital fusion and butterfly vertebrae. There is an associated right paraspinal mass. (C) Axial CT through the lesion shows that it is in direct continuation with the spinal canal through a large ventral bony defect. (D) Axial T_2 and (E) axial T_1 at the level of the lesion demonstrating that the lesion is cystic. (F) Axial T_2 through the bony defect demonstrates the direct continuity of the cyst with the spinal canal. The appearances are in keeping with a neuroenteric cyst. The thoracic cord is also seen to extend through the bony defect. The neural tissue is seen to lie to the left of the neuroenteric cyst. (G) Sagittal T_2 in the right paramidline demonstrating the direct communication with the spinal canal.

signal than cerebrospinal fluid, on T_1 as well as T_2 sequences, but are clearly demarcated from cord substance. Communication with the spinal canal is clearly demonstrated by both CT and MRI (Fig. 4-15).

Dermoid and epidermoid cysts are rounded intradural and sometimes intramedullary lesions. Imaging may demonstrate fat within them and calcification. They may be associated with other forms of dysraphism, and in about 20% a dorsal dermal sinus can be traced running obliquely downwards from the lesion to a skin dimple on the lower back, which may also be a source of intradural sepsis.[20]

Ependymal cysts usually occur with other types of dysraphism. They represent little more than focal dilatations of the central canal of the spinal cord, usually appearing as a swelling near the lumbar enlargement.

Chiari Malformations

These represent a group of abnormalities characterised by dislocation of the hindbrain into the spinal canal. Chiari described four types, but his types III and IV are rare and the Chiari II is seen mainly in the paediatric practice. The Chiari I lesion is not really a malformation at all: it may be acquired in conditions associated with raised intracranial pressure (tumours, venous hypertension), lowered intraspinal pressure (lumbo-peritoneal shunts) and conditions that diminish the volumes of the posterior fossa (craniosynostosis, basilar invagination). It may develop in the first 3 years of life[21] in the absence of any cause other than probable slower growth of the posterior fossa relative to the hindbrain during this period when both are growing most rapidly.

Chiari Type I Lesion (Cerebellar Ectopia)

This is defined as descent of otherwise normal cerebellar hemispheres below the foramen magnum, usually involving the tonsils. However, in about 50% of cases, the medulla oblongata shows elongation of the segment between the pontomedullary junction and dorsal column nuclei with the obex of the fourth ventricle coming to lie in the cervical canal, where it may or may not be overlain by the cerebellar tonsils.

Elongation is sufficient to produce a kink on the posterior surface of the medulla oblongata in about 15%, where the tail of the fourth ventricle rolls down over the upper one or more segments of the spinal cord. The prevalence of Chiari type I lesion in the normal population has been considerably overestimated on MRI, and is probably under 1%.[22]

Chiari Type II Malformations

In these malformations the cerebellum is dysplastic. The inferior vermis is everted rather than inverted so that the nodulus becomes the most inferior part of the cerebellum and the fourth ventricle is reduced to a coronal cleft. The cerebellar herniation then consists mainly of inferior vermis. The medulla oblongata is invariably elongated, usually enough to become kinked. Hydrocephalus and dysplasia of the cerebral hemispheres, cranial vaults and

meninges are frequent. A meningomyelocele is present in 98% or more of cases, and may play an important role in embryogenesis.

These hindbrain abnormalities may be associated with compression and progressive degeneration in parts of the brainstem, cerebellum and upper spinal cord. In Chiari type I malformations, symptoms commonly do not appear until adult life and about 50% of symptomatic cases are associated with syringomyelia. Syringomyelia occurs most commonly when the cerebellar tonsils lie between the neural arches of C1 and C2, whereas cerebellar syndromes predominate when the tonsils lie lower than the neural arch of C2.[23]

In up to 15% of type I lesions, occipitalisation of the atlas and basilar invagination are present.

MRI is by far the best way to demonstrate hindbrain abnormalities, which are present in over 5% of symptomatic cases (Fig. 4-16). However, descent of the cerebellum through the foramen magnum of up to 3 mm is present in up to 20% of normal subjects on mid-sagittal MRI sections due to the shape of the foramen magnum and partial volume effects with the more laterally placed biventral lobules, and MRI in the coronal plane is more reliable (Fig. 4-16).[22]

Meningoceles

Varying degrees of dural ectasia usually accompany the spinal dysraphisms. Both generalised and focal dural ectasia may occur in systemic disorders such as neurofibromatosis, Ehlers–Danlos and Marfan's syndromes. It may occur in erosive arthropathies, especially ankylosing spondylitis,[24] where focal ectasia sometimes forms pockets or saccules invaginating into the walls of the spinal canal, including the vertebral bodies and neural arches. Such lesions also occur idiopathically.

Anterior Sacral Meningocele

This lesion consists of a unilocular, complex lobular or even multilocular presacral cystic mass, containing CSF, which communicates with the intraspinal subarachnoid space.

There is a large usually eccentric anterior defect in the lower part of the sacrum, and the sacral canal is expanded. Varying degrees of sacral and coccygeal agenesis may be associated. On plain radiographs, the eccentric anterior sacral defect gives the remaining part of the sacrum a pathognomonic scimitar appearance. The pelvic mass may be shown by US, CT or MRI, the latter invariably demonstrating communications with the sacral canal (Fig. 4-17).

Occult intrasacral meningocele is a variant of this condition. The sacral canal is expanded by a meningocele that lies below the normal level of termination of the thecal sac. There is no anterior sacral defect and no intrapelvic extension.

Lateral Thoracic Meningocele

This lesion commonly presents as a paravertebral mass on chest radiography. It is commonly solitary and usually is found on the right; 70–85% of lesions are associated with neurofibromatosis. There is typically an angular

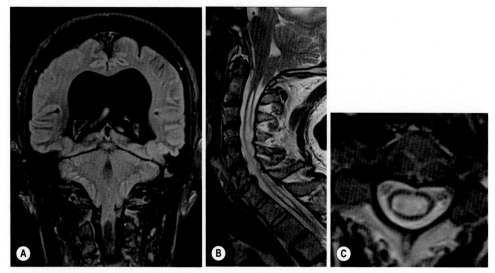

FIGURE 4-16 ■ **Chiari I malformation.** (A) Coronal FLAIR demonstrating bitonsilar herniation. Note the secondary hydrocephalus. (B) Sagittal T₂ demonstrating the Chiari malformation and an associated extensive cervical syrinx cavity. (C) Axial T₂ showing syrinx cavity of CSF density.

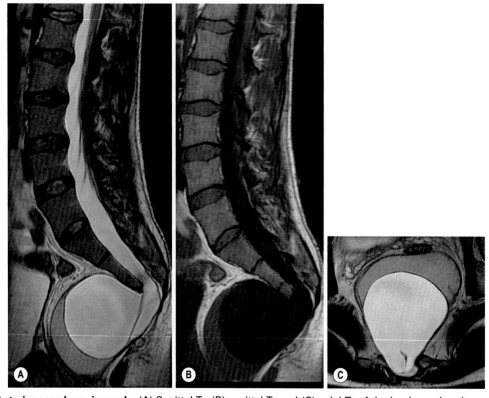

FIGURE 4-17 ■ **Anterior sacral meningocele.** (A) Sagittal T₂, (B) sagittal T₁ and (C) axial T₂ of the lumbar spine demonstrating a large presacral cystic mass that is in direct continuation with the vertebral canal through an anterior vertebral defect. Note the agenesis of the coccyx and the lower sacrum.

kyphoscoliosis towards the side of the meningocele, and pressure erosion of the margins of the relevant intervertebral foramen is evident.

Anterior Thoracic Meningocele with Ventral Herniation of Spinal Cord

This is an increasingly recognised condition very occasionally providing explanation for an otherwise unexplained chronic thoracic myelopathy in adults.[25] It is most readily recognised on mid-sagittal MRI of the thoracic spine, where the spinal cord is displaced anteriorly in contact with a vertebral body at or very near an intervertebral disc, commonly at about T6. The meningocele may not be easy to show on axial images. Appearances are often misinterpreted as an intradural arachnoid cyst displacing the spinal cord anteriorly, from which the condition needs to be distinguished.

Intraspinal Arachnoid Cyst

Extradural arachnoid cysts arise from defects in the dura mater, either congenital or inflammatory (e.g. ankylosing spondylitis); intradural arachnoid cysts arise from arachnoidal duplications or spinal arachnoiditis. Symptoms of pain or neurological disability may arise when the spinal cord or cauda equina is compressed, bearing in mind that size and intracystic pressure may vary considerably. Occasionally, the spinal cord or roots herniate through a dural defect and become entrapped. Plain radiographs may show expansion of the spinal canal when the cyst is extradural. MRI shows these lesions well (Fig. 4-18). Signal from fluid in the cyst, and often from the subarachnoid space below it, is usually higher than from CSF elsewhere due to reduced mobility. Effects on the spinal cord, namely compression and rarely myelomalacia or syringomyelia, are shown. Small herniations of neural tissue through the dural defects may require thin imaging sections and high-resolution imaging techniques to show them. Aspiration and drainage of arachnoid cysts compressing the spinal cord may be

accompanied by immediate and dramatic improvement in clinical condition.[26]

Care must be exercised not to overdiagnose intradural arachnoid cysts in the thoracic region. The retromedullary subarachnoid space in the thoracic spine is commonly wide, and partly loculated by usually incomplete septae; the spinal cord usually is closely applied to the anterior margin of the bony canal and may have a flattened appearance over an exaggerated kyphosis.

Perineural arachnoid cysts (Tarlov cysts) occur commonly in the sacrum, especially on the second sacral root. They can be large, multiple and are often associated with eccentric pressure erosion of the sacral canal and are well shown by MRI. Clinical significance, even of large cysts, is doubtful.[27]

Syringomyelia

The term 'syringomyelia' describes conditions in which there is a cavity within the spinal cord, lined mainly by glial tissue and containing fluid that is similar or identical

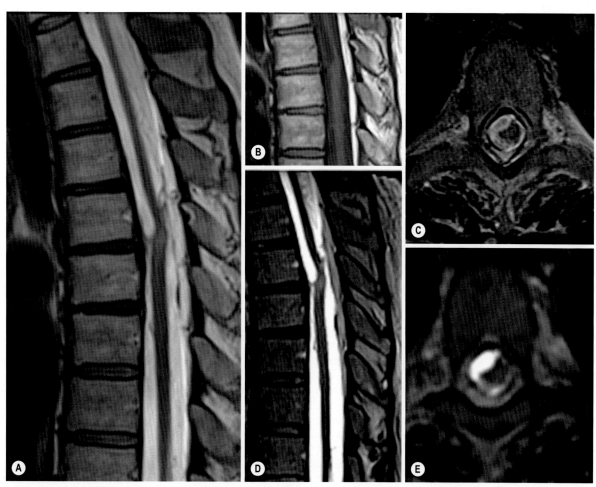

FIGURE 4-18 ■ Intraspinal arachnoid cyst. (A) Sagittal T_2, (B) sagittal T_1 and (C) axial T_2 of the thoracic spine demonstrating an abnormal appearance to the mid-thoracic cord, which is moulded and displaced to the left by a right anterior intradural extramedullary lesion of CSF signal intensity. There is focal volume loss and subtle intrinsic signal change within the cord at this level in keeping with focal myelomalacia from compression. The conventional T_2 (A and C) images demonstrate CSF flow-related artefact in the lesion (focal areas of signal drop). This artefact is not present on (D) sagittal CISS and (E) axial CISS images, which demonstrate the lesion more clearly.

with CSF. It is associated with a number of distinct pathological processes, including cerebellar ectopia and trauma.[28] Whatever the cause, the cavity seems capable of propagating, probably due to hydrodynamic forces, into normal cord tissue. Usually it involves many segments or the whole spinal cord, but sometimes smaller isolated cavities are found confined to only a few spinal segments, often referred to as fusiform syrinx. The cervical cord is involved most often, although occasionally only the thoracic cord. Only about 10% of cysts extend cranial to C2, where they split into two or deviate to right or left in a plane ventral to the floor of the fourth ventricle. Small cavities usually involve the bases of the posterior columns, and commonly the central cord canal for part of their extent; larger cavities are associated with more extensive loss of cord substance. Double cavities are sometimes present and individual cavities may be multilocular. The spinal cord is enlarged in about 80% of cases, normal in size in 10% and diffusely atrophic in 10%. The size of the spinal cord may vary in response to posture and respiration. Size variation usually is not associated with changes in clinical state, nor does the severity of clinical disability relate to the size of the cyst and remaining cord substance.[29]

Between 70 and 90% of cases of syringomyelia are associated with cerebellar ectopia, the cerebellar tonsils usually lying at the level of C1 or between C1 and C2 (Fig. 4-16).[23] It is postulated that intermittent obstruction of the outlets of the fourth ventricle and of CSF flow across the foramen magnum, combined with a patent communication between the fourth ventricle and the central canal of the spinal cord, together produce secondary degeneration of cord substance by causing intermittent distension of the central canal but alternative hypotheses exist.[30] The term syringohydromyelia is often used for this type of cord cavitation.

Other causes of cavitation of the spinal cord can result in appearances indistinguishable from syringohydromyelia. These include intramedullary tumours, spinal cord trauma and inflammatory processes discussed earlier in this chapter, which can result in colliquative necrosis (myelomalacia), which may organise into cavities that propagate into normal cord substance. Finally in about 10–20% of patients with spinal cord cavities, no cause or association can be found.

Syringomyelia and its cause are well demonstrated by MRI, which shows a well-circumscribed cavity of a similar signal to CSF on T_1 and T_2 sequences (Fig. 4-16). Pulsatile cysts may show flow-related signal changes.[31] Dynamic MRI, using phase-contrast techniques, has been used to study CSF movement, especially at foramen magnum level.[32]

A moderate correlation is found between the presence and location of the cavity on MRI and clinical features, but *not* between clinical severity and size of the syrinx relative to remaining cord substance, *or* with its degree of distension.[33–35] MRI is good for monitoring the mechanical success of operative strategies,[36] of which three are in current use, the third being new and controversial, deriving from an alternative theory of causation: (A) foramen magnum decompression; (B) syringosubarachnoid, peritoneal or pleural shunting; and (C) lumbo-peritoneal shunting.[37,38] All seem equally effective in obtaining, and generally maintaining, collapse of the syrinx in 70–80% of cases. Unfortunately, however, clinical outcome and extension of cord cavitation on interval images seem to bear no relation to whether the cavity remains collapsed.[36]

NEURODEGENERATIVE AND METABOLIC DISEASES

Motor Neuron Disease (MND)

This condition comprises a group of progressive neurodegenerative diseases affecting the upper and lower motor neurons of the brain and spinal cord. They can be classified according to the type of motor neuron it affects. In amyotrophic lateral sclerosis (ALS) both upper and lower neurons are affected at two or more levels; progressive muscular atrophy (PMA) involves only the lower motor neurons, whilst primary lateral sclerosis (PLS) involves only upper motor neurons. Rarely, the disease is restricted to the bulbar muscles, secondary to disease affecting the motor nuclei in the medulla, when it is termed progressive bulbar palsy (PBP).

ALS, also known as Lou Gehrig disease, is the most common of the motor neurodegenerative diseases and almost all cases evolve to this. Most cases are sporadic, with only approximately 5–10% being familial, inherited in an autosomal dominant pattern.[39] Most commonly the presentation is a mixed pattern of hand weakness and atrophy of the intrinsic hand muscles, together with hyperreflexia and ataxia reflecting lower and upper motor neuron involvement, respectively. Limb fasciculations are common. With disease progression comes weakness and atrophy of the lower limb, dysarthria, dysphagia and tongue fasciculations. Prognosis is poor, with death from respiratory failure.

MRI plays a role in excluding other diagnoses, such as MS or radiculopathy, but can be normal. Positive MRI findings are of symmetrical T_2 hyperintensity in the lateral columns, best appreciated on axial imaging,[40] correlating well with histopathological findings affecting primarily the lateral corticospinal tracts.

Spinal Muscular Atrophy (SMA)

This is a large group of genetically associated autosomal recessive neuromuscular disorders, characterised by loss of the spinal lower motor neurons in the anterior horns with no sensory or pyramidal tract involvement. The genetic defects associated with SMA types I–III are localised on chromosome 5q11.2-13.3.[41] The international SMA consortium meeting recognises four distinct subtypes based on age of onset: (A) type I, acute infantile form; (B) type II, chronic infantile or intermediate form; (C) type III, juvenile form; and (D) type IV, adult form.[42] MRI may reveal focal atrophy of the cervical cord with an associated small area of T_2 hyperintensity. These findings are non-specific and associated with focal myelomalacia from other causes, for example following trauma.

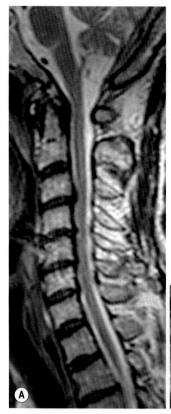

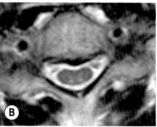

FIGURE 4-19 ■ **Subacute combined degeneration of the spinal cord (SCD) in a 60-year-old man after gastrectomy.** (A) Sagittal T₂ showing linear high signal intensity in the cervical spinal cord extending over two segments, without associated cord swelling. (B) Typical bilateral dorsal hyperintensities are demonstrated on axial T₂.

Spinocerebellar Ataxia

This term encompasses a large group of progressive inherited neurodegenerative disorders characterised by ataxia and poor coordination of hand, speech and eye movements which are progressive. They are classified by mode of inheritance and the causative gene. The most common of the autosomal dominant group is spinocerebellar degeneration, itself consisting of different subtypes. Friedreich's ataxia is the commonest of the autosomal recessive forms.

Friedreich's Ataxia (FRDA)

This is the most common inherited ataxia. It is caused by mutations in the frataxin gene, causing loss of large primary neurons in the dorsal root ganglia, sensory fibres in peripheral nerves, degeneration of the posterior and lateral columns of the spinal cord and atrophy of the cerebellar dentate nucleus. It presents with progressive limb and gait ataxia, dysarthria, loss of position and vibration senses and areflexia.

MRI of the spine demonstrates thinning of the cervical spinal cord, particularly in the anterior posterior dimension. There is also frequently intramedullary T₂ hyperintensity, which is symmetrical within the posterior or lateral columns of the spinal cord.[43]

Subacute Combined Degeneration of the Spinal Cord (SCD)

This is a progressive myelopathy presenting with sensory symptoms in the context of dietary deficiency of vitamin B₁₂ or co-proteins. Vitamin B₁₂ deficiency can be due to malabsorption syndromes, previous gastrectomy, pernicious anemia and dietary deficiencies (e.g. in strict vegetarians). The lateral and dorsal spinal cord columns are affected, and improvement is often only partial after treatment. A typical MR imaging finding is a linear hyperintensity on sagittal T₂ located bilateral dorsally in the cord (Fig. 4-19) that regresses on treatment. Lesions, which are most often seen between C2 and C5, may enhance after IV contrast medium. However, MRI may also remain negative.[44]

FURTHER READING

Agosta F, Filippi M. MRI of spinal cord in multiple sclerosis. J Neuroimaging 2007;17(Suppl 1):46S–9S.

Borchers AT, Gershwin ME. Transverse myelitis. Autoimmun Rev 2012;11:231–48.

Bot JC, Barkhof F. Spinal-cord MRI in multiple sclerosis: conventional and nonconventional MR techniques. Neuroimaging Clin N Am 2009;19:81–99.

Lycklama G, Thompson A, Filippi M, et al. Spinal-cord MRI in multiple sclerosis. Lancet Neurol 2003;2:555–62.

McKeon A, Lennon VA, Lotze T, et al. CNS aquaporin-4 autoimmunity in children. Neurology 2008;71:93–100.

Pavone P, Pettoello-Mantovano M, Le Pira A, et al. Acute disseminated encephalomyelitis: a long-term prospective study and meta-analysis. Neuropediatrics 2010;41:246–55.

Pittock SJ, Lennon VA, Krecke K, et al. Brain abnormalities in neuromyelitis optica. Arch Neurol 2006;63:390–6.

Sellner J, Lüthi N, Bühler R, et al. Acute partial transverse myelitis: risk factors for conversion to multiple sclerosis. Eur J Neurol 2008;15:398–405.

Thomas T, Branson HM, Verhey LH, et al. Demographic, clinical, and magnetic resonance imaging (MRI) features of transverse myelitis in children. J Child Neurol 2011;27(1):11–21.

Wender M. Acute disseminated encephalomyelitis. J Neuroimmunol 2011;231:92–9.

Weinshenker BG, Wingerchuk DM. Neuromyelitis optica: clinical syndrome and the NMO-IgG autoantibody marker. Curr Top Microbiol Immunol 2008;318:343–56.

Wingerchuk DM, Lennon VA, Pittock SJ, et al. Revised diagnostic criteria for neuromyelitis optica. Neurology 2006;66:1485–9.

REFERENCES

1. Brilot F, Dale RC, Selter RC, et al. Antibodies to native myelin oligodendrocyte glycoprotein in children with inflammatory demyelinating central nervous system disease. Ann Neurol 2009;66:833–42.

2. Transverse Myelitis Consortium Working Group. Proposed diagnostic criteria and nosology of acute transverse myelitis. Neurology 2002;59:499–505.

3. Lennon VA, Wingerchuk DM, Kryzer TJ, et al. A serum autoantibody marker of neuromyelitis optica: distinction from multiple sclerosis. Lancet 2004;364:2106–12.

4. Krampla W, Aboul-Enein F, Jecel J, et al. Spinal cord lesions in patients with neuromyelitis optica: a retrospective long-term MRI follow-up study. Eur Radiol 2009;19:2535–43.

5. Kim W, Kim SH, Kim HJ. New insights into neuromyelitis optica. J Clin Neurol 2011;7:115–27.

6. Kim JE, Kim SM, Ahn SW, et al. Brain abnormalities in neuromyelitis optica. J Neurol Sci 2011;302:43–8.

7. Birnbaum J, Petri M, Thompson R, et al. Distinct subtypes of myelitis in systemic lupus erythematosus. Arthritis Rheum 2009;60:3378–87.

8. Jacobs BC, Koga M, van Rijs W, et al. Subclass IgG to motor gangliosides related to infection and clinical course in Guillain-Barré syndrome. J Neuroimmunol 2008;194(1–2):181–90.

9. Kendall BE, Logue V. Spinal epidural angiomatous malformations draining into intrathecal veins. Neuroradiology 1997;13:181–9.

10. Gilbertson JR, Miller GM, Goldman MS, et al. Spinal dural arteriovenous fistulas: MR and myelographic findings. Am J Neuroradiol 1995;16:2049–57.

11. Farb RI, Kim JK, Willinsky RA, et al. Spinal dural arteriovenous fistula localization with a technique of first-pass gadolinium-enhanced MR angiography: initial experience. Radiology 2002;222:843–50.

12. Willinsky R, Lasjaunias P, Terbrugge K, Hurth M. Spinal angiography in the investigation of spinal arteriovenous fistula. A protocol with application to the venous phase. Neuroradiology 1990;32:114–16.

13. Van Dijk JM, TerBrugge KG, Willinsky RA, et al. Multidisciplinary management of spinal dural arteriovenous fistulas: clinical presentation and long-term follow-up in 49 patients. Stroke 2002;33:1578–83.

14. Andres RH, Barth A, Guzman R, et al. Endovascular and surgical treatment of spinal dural arteriovenous fistulas. Neuroradiology 2008;50:869–76.

15. Krings T, Thron AK, Geibprasert A, et al. Endovascular management of spinal vascular malformations. Neurosurg Rev 2010;33(1):1–9.

16. Willinsky RA. Spinal cord arteriovenous malformations. In: Marks MP, Do HM, editors. Endovascular and Percutaneous Therapy of the Brain and Spine. Philadelphia: Lippincott Williams & Wilkins; 2002. pp. 415–48.

17. Ogilvy CS, Louis DN, Ojemann RG. Intramedullary cavernous angiomas of the spinal cord: clinical presentation, pathological features, and surgical management. Neurosurgery 1992;31(2):219–29.

18. David KM, Copp AJ, Stevens JM, et al. Split cervical spinal cord with Klippel–Feil syndrome: seven cases. Brain 1996;119(6):1859–72.

19. Brooks BS, Duval ER, El Hammal P, et al. Neuroimaging features of neuroenteric cysts: analysis of nine cases and review of the literature. Am J Neuroradiol 1993;14:735–46.

20. Rogg JM, Benzil DL, Haas RL, Knucky NW. Intramedullary abscess, an unusual manifestation of a dermal sinus. Am J Neuroradiol 1993;14:1393–5.

21. Huang PP, Constantine S. Acquired Chiari I malformations. J Neurosurg 1994;80:1099–102.

22. Savy L, Stevens JM, Taylor DJ, Knedall BE. Apparent cerebellar ectopia: a reappraisal using volumetric MRI. Neuroradiology 1994;6:360–3.

23. Stevens JM, Serva W, Kendall BE, et al. Chiari malformation in adults: relation of morphological aspects to clinical features and operative outcome. J Neurol Neurosurg Psychiatry 1993;56:1072–7.

24. Young A, Dixon AK, Getty J, et al. Cauda equina syndrome complicating ankylosing spondylitis: use of electromyography and computerised tomography in diagnosis. Ann Rheum Dis 1981;40:317–22.

25. Walters MR, Stears JC, Osborn AG. Transdural spinal cord herniation: imaging and clinical spectra. Am J Neuroradiol 1998;19:1335–6.

26. Stevens JM, Kendall BE, Davis C, Crockard HA. Percutaneous insertion of the spinal end of a cystoperitoneal shunt as definitive treatment to relieve spinal cord compression from spinal arachnoid cyst. Neuroradiology 1987;29:190–5.

27. Van de Kelft E, Van Vyve M. Sacral meningeal cysts and perineal pain. Lancet 1993;341:500–1.

28. Potter K, Saifuddin A. MRI of chronic spinal cord injury. Br J Radiol 2003;76:347–52.

29. Grant R, Hadley DM, MacPherson P. Syringomyelia: cyst measurement by magnetic resonance imaging and comparison with symptoms, signs and disability. J Neurol Neurosurg Psychiatry 1987;50:1008–14.

30. Williams B. Pathogenesis of syringomyelia. Lancet 1972;i:142–3.

31. Enzmann DR, O'Donohue J, Rubin JB, et al. CSF pulsations within non-neoplastic spinal cord cysts. Am J Neuroradiol 1987;8:517–25.

32. Quencer RM, Donovan-Post MJ, Hinks RS. Cine MR in the evaluation of normal and abnormal CSF flow: intracranial and intraspinal studies. Neuroradiology 1990;32:371–91.

33. Ulmer JL, Mathews VP, Elster AD, et al. Lumbar spondylolysis without spondylolisthesis. Am J Roentgenol 1997;169:233–7.

34. Stevens JM, Olney JS, Kendall BE. Post-traumatic cystic and noncystic myelopathy. Neuroradiology 1985;27:48–56.

35. Sherman JL, Berkovich AJ, Citrin CM. The MR appearances of syringomyelia: new observations. Am J Neuroradiol 1986;7:985–95.

36. Vaquero J, Martinez R, Arlas A. Syringomyelia-Chiari complex. Magnetic resonance imaging and clinical evaluation of surgical treatment. J Neurosurg 1990;73:14–18.

37. Milhorat TH, Johnson WD, Miller JI, et al. Surgical treatment of syringomyelia based on magnetic resonance imaging criteria. Neurosurgery 1992;31:231–42.

38. Vissilouthis J, Panadreon A, Anagnostasas S. Theco-peritoneal shunt for syringomyelia: Report of three cases. Neurosurgery 1993;33:324–8.

39. Armon C, Epidemiology of ALS/MND. In: Shaw P, Strong M, editors. Motor Neuron Disorders. Elsevier Sciences; 2003. pp. 167–206.

40. Thorpe JW, Moseley IF, Hawkes CH, et al. Brain and spinal cord MRI in motor neuron disease. J Neurol Neurosurg Psychiatry 1996;61(3):314–17.

41. Brzustowicz LM, Lehner T, Castilla LH, et al. Genetic mapping of chronic childhood-onset spinal muscular atrophy to chromosome 5q11.2-13.3. Nature 1990;344(6266):540–1.

42. Munsat TL, Davies KE. International SMA consortium meeting. (26–28 June 1992, Bonn, Germany) Neuromuscul Disord 1992;2(5–6):423–8.

43. Mascalchi M, Salvi F, Piacentini S, et al. Friedreich's ataxia: MR findings involving the cervical portion of the spinal cord. Am J Roentgenol 1994;16:187–91.

44. Locatelli ER, Laurena R, Ballard P, Mark AS. MRI in vitamin B_{12} deficiency myelopathy. Can Neurol Sci 1999;26:60–3.

CHAPTER 5

POSTOPERATIVE SPINE

Tomasz Matys • Nasim Sheikh-Bahaei • Jonathan H. Gillard

CHAPTER OUTLINE

INTRODUCTION

PRINCIPLES OF SPINAL SURGERY

IMAGING TECHNIQUES IN POSTOPERATIVE
SPINE

INTRAOPERATIVE AND PERIOPERATIVE
COMPLICATIONS

EARLY COMPLICATIONS

LATE COMPLICATIONS

IMAGE-GUIDED PERCUTANEOUS CEMENT BONE
AUGMENTATION

INTRODUCTION

Imaging plays an important role in the assessment of the postoperative spine. The main objectives of imaging are to evaluate the alignment of the spinal column, the position of implants and the status of fusion or fracture healing, and to demonstrate potential complications in case of persistent or new postoperative symptoms.[1,2] Postsurgical appearances may be complex, and knowledge of indications for surgery, type of the procedure, hardware and biomaterials used and pertinent clinical information is essential to avoid misinterpretation.[3] In this chapter we discuss principles of spinal surgery and briefly review its potential complications with emphasis on these most often encountered in radiological practice.

PRINCIPLES OF SPINAL SURGERY

The goals of spinal surgery can be broadly categorised into three main groups:
1. Decompression of neural structures, for example by removal of herniated disc material, widening of a stenosed spinal canal, or removal of a displaced fracture fragment.
2. Stabilisation of the spinal column in order to reduce pain caused by motion segments, ensure stability after a fracture or resection of spinal elements, prevent progression of deformity, or reduce its degree.
3. Excision of spinal tumours.

In order to achieve decompression, several surgical techniques are employed, usually in combination.[1,4] Removal of intervertebral disc material is performed by discectomy or minimally invasive microdiscectomy; access to herniated disc may require removal of the margins of the lamina (laminotomy), unilateral laminar resection (hemi-laminectomy) and resection of the ligamentum flavum (flavectomy). Techniques used in spinal canal decompression include laminoplasty (osteotomy of one lamina with contralateral partial osteotomy to allow formation of a unilateral gap), bilateral laminectomy with the removal of the posterior elements and deroofing of the spinal canal and/or facetectomy (excision of a part or entire facet joint). Neural foraminal decompression is achieved by foraminotomy. More extensive techniques used in the management of traumatic fractures and primary or metastatic spinal tumours include resection of one or both pedicles (pediculectomy), vertebral body (corpectomy) or entire vertebra (vertebrectomy).

Stabilisation can be the primary goal of surgery, or can be performed in combination with decompressive or excision procedures that impair spine stability. In the majority of cases, a stabilisation procedure consists of instrumentation and bone grafting. Types of fixation devices used include translaminar or facet screws, and transpedicular screws in conjunction with rods, plates, hooks, wires or clamps.[1] It is important to realise that metalwork, although usually left in place indefinitely, is only relied upon for temporary support until uninterrupted osseous union is achieved. Bone fusion can be promoted by a variety of graft materials.[5] Autologous bone grafts are most often harvested from the iliac crest, another part of the spine, or for purely cortical bone, from the tibia or fibula. Ground-up (morselised) cancellous bone chips are used to promote osteogenesis (Fig. 5-1A), while cortical bone is used for structural support (Figs. 5-1B, C). Allograft bone substitutes are obtained from the tissue bank and include femoral rings, fibular struts and bone chips that can be used on their own or to supplement allografts. Synthetic graft substitutes include recombinant bone morphogenetic protein (BMP), demineralised bone matrix (DBX) and ceramics

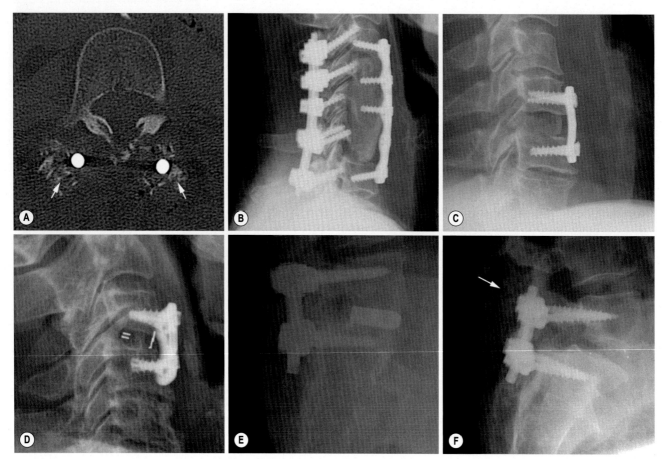

FIGURE 5-1 ■ (A) Axial CT image showing morselised bone chips (arrows) in a patient with lumbar fixation. (B) Lateral radiograph of the cervical spine showing autologous bone graft from iliac crest used for structural support in a patient with C4–C6 corpectomies for chordoma treatment. Note anterior plate and posterior fixation with pedicular screws and rods spanning C3–C7 levels. (C) Inter-body cortical autologous bone graft in a patient after anterior cervical discectomy and fusion (ACDF). (D) Synthetic radiolucent interbody cage used in ACDF; note radiopaque cage markers in the intervertebral space. (E) Lateral radiograph of the lumbar spine in a patient after posterior lumbar interbody fusion (PLIF) with radiopaque cage. (F) Patient with transforaminal lumbar interbody fusion (TFLI) using radiolucent cage; radiopaque cage markers are visible as dots in the intervertebral space. Also note bone chips posterior to the fixation hardware (arrow).

(tricalcium phosphate, hydroxyapatite or calcium sulphate), available in a variety of forms and consistencies. Increasingly, synthetic cages[6] manufactured from metal (titanium or tantalum) or non-metallic radiolucent material such as carbon composite polymers, polyetheretherketone (PEEK) or bioabsorbable polylactic acid (PLA) are used instead of cortical bone for structural support in vertebral interbody fusion procedures (Figs. 5-1D–F). Such implants provide immediate load-bearing capacity while fusion occurs in their core packed with autologous cancellous bone, allograft or synthetic bone substitute.

Spinal surgery can be performed from anterior, posterior or combined approaches. An anterior approach is primarily used in the cervical spine for procedures such as anterior cervical discectomy and fusion (ACDF), and anterior instrumentation for corpectomy, peg fracture fixation with anterior screws, cervical foraminotomy and disc replacement. The traditional open anterior approach in the lumbar spine has been more difficult, but with increasing use of minimally invasive surgery (MIS)[7] and endoscopic surgical techniques this route is now more frequently used, for example for anterior lumbar

interbody fusion (ALIF). A posterior approach is used in discectomy, foraminotomy, spinal canal decompression, various types of fixation using pedicle, translaminar or transfacet screws, and insertion of interspinous spacers, as well as posterior lumbar interbody fusion (PLIF) and transforaminal lumbar interbody fusion (TLIF). Anterior and posterior approaches can be combined in '360° fusion' procedures in which anterior interbody fusion is accompanied by posterior stabilisation with translaminar or pedicle screws, and facet joint or intertransversal fixation. Scoliosis correction surgery may require an anterior or posterior approach, depending on individual anatomical considerations and involved spinal segment.[1,2,7]

IMAGING TECHNIQUES IN POSTOPERATIVE SPINE

Plain radiographs are commonly used in routine follow-up of the instrumented spine to assess hardware migration, loosening or breakage. Radiography is inexpensive, is quick to perform and is the only technique allowing imaging with the patient in an upright position. Antero-posterior and lateral projections can be supplemented with dynamic flexion and extension views to assess motion at the fusion site and adjacent segments suggestive of pseudoarthrosis and instability. Serial radiographs may be helpful in demonstrating subtle changes in implant positioning.

More precise evaluation of implant position, alignment and integrity and fusion status is provided by CT. As the majority of implants are made of titanium, which has lower radiographic density than steel, beam hardening artefacts are generally minimal. The amount of artefact is further reduced by using helical acquisition (which also enables multiplanar reformats), high tube voltage and current, narrow collimation, thin sections and low pitch. Reconstruction with smooth or standard kernel may be preferable as bone kernel algorithm can accentuate artefacts. Average intensity projection (AIP) may be helpful in assessing hardware integrity.[8] In non-implant-related complications and non-instrumented spine, CT has been largely superseded by MRI, but may still play a role in patients with claustrophobia or contraindications to entering the magnet.

MRI is the technique of choice in non-hardware-related complications due to its ability to image soft tissue and neural structures, and conspicuity of contrast enhancement. It may demonstrate early complications such as haemorrhage, infection or dural leaks, and helps differentiate causes of persistent or recurrent symptoms.[3,9] Protocols vary depending on institutional experience, especially with regards to routine use of fat suppression and gadolinium contrast medium—while some authors advocate a contrast-enhanced T1 sequence in all postoperative patients,[3] other institutions rely on unenhanced T2-weighted images for routine assessment.[10] Early postoperative appearances can be difficult to interpret and misleading due to signal changes in intervertebral disc, endplates and epidural soft tissues that may mimic the appearances of disc herniation and lead to false impression of residual disc material. Bone removal can be difficult to assess on T2-weighted images, and T1-weighted sections are better suited for this purpose.[3,9] The presence of spinal implants is not a contraindication to MRI. Susceptibility artefacts from metallic implants are less problematic at lower field strengths and can be minimised by avoiding

gradient-echo sequences, using fast spin-echo techniques, high receiver bandwidth, small voxel size, short TE and anterior-to-posterior frequency-encoding direction.[11]

INTRAOPERATIVE AND PERIOPERATIVE COMPLICATIONS

Intra- and perioperative complications can be related to injury of structures and organs during approach to the surgical site, or to surgical technique including hardware misplacement. For example, an anterior approach to the cervical spine puts at risk the recurrent laryngeal nerve, with transient or permanent palsy due to excessive retraction or transection. Injury to vertebral artery is a rare but potentially catastrophic event. The most dreaded complication is the spinal cord injury; direct iatrogenic trauma is uncommon, but spinal cord function may be impaired by patient positioning or intraoperative hypotension, especially if there is a pre-existing cord compression or contusion. Paraspinal visceral structures that are at risk of injury during approach or by screws of excessive length or aberrant course include trachea, oesophagus, lung, pleura, thoracic duct, aorta and great vessels, heart, ureter, peritoneum and bowel.[1,7] Imaging in cases of damage to these structures should be tailored to the clinical scenario and specific organ and injury pattern.

Hardware-related complications in the perioperative period are mostly related to misplaced transpedicular screws. CT is the best technique for demonstrating screw placement, which should be wholly contained within the respective pedicles and covered by cortical bone from all sides (Figs. 5-2A, B); the screw tip should approach, but not breach, the anterior cortex of the vertebral body. Misplaced screws (Figs. 5-2C, D) may impinge on the spinal canal or neural foramen, threatening the spinal cord, cauda equina or exiting nerve roots. The reported rate of misplacement is high and may exceed 40%;[1] however, clinically significant impingement or injury of neural structures is less common. The incidence of radiculopathy is reported at 7% and the nerve root is most at risk of injury or irritation if the medial or inferior border of the pedicle is violated. The need for screw removal or revision is dictated by neurological symptoms, taking into account the degree of misplacement.

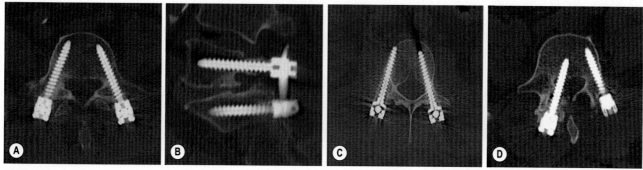

FIGURE 5-2 ■ Axial CT image (A) and sagittal oblique reformat (B) demonstrating satisfactory placement of transpedicular screws. (C) Misplaced right screw coursing laterally to the pedicle. (D) Misplaced right screw coursing medially to the pedicle through the lateral recess.

EARLY COMPLICATIONS

Early complications of spinal surgery include haemorrhage, cerebrospinal fluid (CSF) leak and infection.[1,7,9]

Postoperative haemorrhage is uncommon (less than 1% of patients) and usually occurs in the immediate postoperative period. In the cervical spine, expanding neck wound haematoma can lead to airway compression and is a surgical emergency;[12] the role of imaging is limited as the diagnosis is usually clinical and urgent wound exploration should be performed without delay. Symptoms of spinal cord or cauda equina compression in the early postoperative period are suspicious for epidural haematoma.[1] Small amounts of asymptomatic epidural haemorrhage are present in most procedures involving the spinal canal, but symptomatic haematoma requiring evacuation occurs in less than 0.5% of patients on average, being the highest in the thoracic spine at 4.5%.[13] MRI is

the technique of choice for identifying the extent of haemorrhage and compression of neural structures. Findings include an epidural mass with T1 signal dependent on age of the haematoma (iso- or hypointense in acute haemorrhage, hyperintense in chronic haematoma) and heterogeneously hyperintense on T2-weighted sequences, with no contrast enhancement (Fig. 5-3).

CSF leak is an equally uncommon complication of spinal surgery, occurring as a result of unrecognised or improperly repaired dural breach. Extravasation of CSF into surrounding tissues leads to formation of a pseudomeningocele. CSF can also egress through the surgical wound or drain track, resulting in a cutaneous CSF fistula. MRI is an investigation of choice as it readily demonstrates fluid signal intensity collections in the paraspinal soft tissues related to the thecal sac; communication with the thecal sac can sometimes be visualised. There is no enhancement, or thin peripheral enhancement only (Fig. 5-4). Pseudomeningocele needs to be

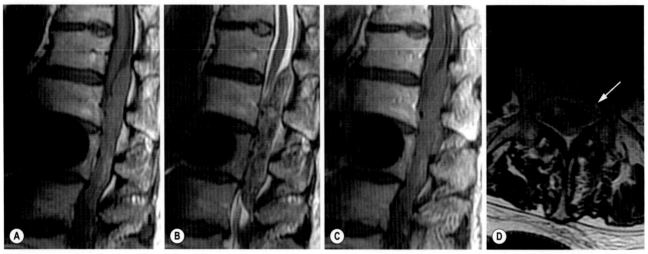

FIGURE 5-3 ■ **Epidural haematoma.** Sagittal MRI images demonstrate epidural mass slightly hyperintense to spinal cord on T1-weighted images (A) and of heterogeneous signal on T2 sequence (B), with no enhancement following gadolinium administration (C). Roots of cauda equina are displaced anteriorly and to the left (arrow) and compressed (D).

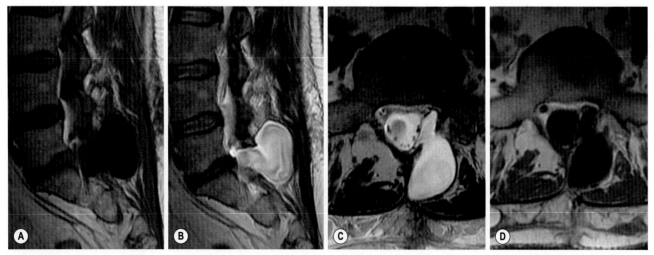

FIGURE 5-4 ■ **Pseudomeningocele in a patient after left S1 nerve root decompression procedure.** Sagittal T1-weighted (A) and T2-weighted (B) images demonstrate fluid intensity collection in the posterior paraspinal soft tissues. Axial T2 image (C) shows fluid collection related to the extradural part of S1 nerve root and extending through flavectomy defect to the left of the spinous process. Post-contrast T1 image (D) shows lack of enhancement.

differentiated from true meningocele with expansion of the dura through the surgical spinal canal defect, postoperative haematoma and abscess. A CT myelogram can be helpful in localising the exact site of extravasation and outlining the fistulous track. Pseudomeningocele may be associated with signs of intracranial hypotension (CSF leakage syndrome) such as dural thickening and enhancement, 'sagging' midbrain, tonsillar herniation, venous distension, pituitary gland enlargement and subdural haematomas or hygromas.[2]

Postoperative infections complicate 0.2–3% of spinal procedures and include a spectrum of wound infections, discitis, vertebral osteomyelitis, and epidural abscess, which can occur in isolation or combined. Most cases are caused by direct staphylococcal infection and should be suspected in all patients with persistent back pain

occurring weeks to months after surgery. The white cell count often remains within normal limits but erythrocyte sedimentation ratio and C-reactive protein levels are elevated. In infection limited to the surgical wound there are no intervertebral disc or vertebral body signal changes (Fig. 5-5). Features of intervertebral disc involvement on MRI include loss of disc height, T1 hypointensity with T2 hyperintensity, and contrast enhancement of the intervertebral disc space; similar signal changes and enhancement in adjacent endplates indicate extension of disc infection and vertebral osteomyelitis (Fig. 5-6). An associated paraspinal abscess appears as enhancing soft tissue with areas of fluid intensity; thick enhancing rim and surrounding oedema can also be seen. The diagnosis of spondylodiscitis in the early postoperative period may be difficult as intervertebral space and endplate changes

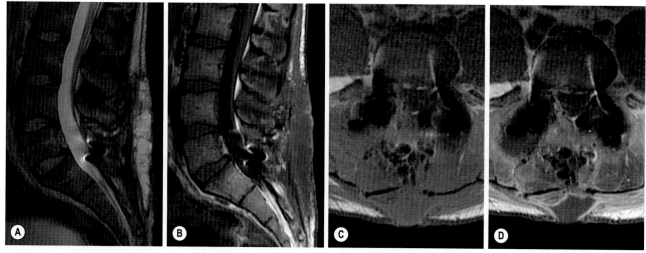

FIGURE 5-5 ■ **Wound infection in a patient with posterior lumbar fixation.** Sagittal T1 (A) and T2 (B) images demonstrate complex mass in the posterior paraspinal and subcutaneous soft tissues. Axial T1-weighted images before (C) and after administration of gadolinium (D) demonstrate avid ring enhancement around fluid collection in subcutaneous soft tissues close to the skin surface, and diffuse enhancement in the paraspinal soft tissues. Note normal signal intensity in intervertebral discs and vertebral bodies.

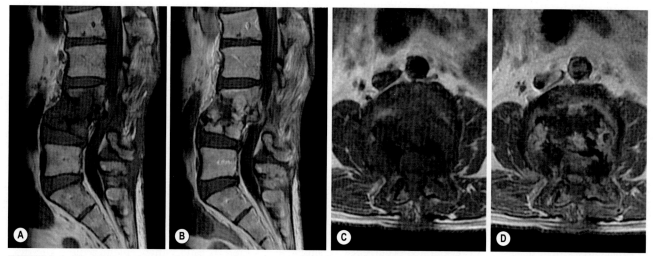

FIGURE 5-6 ■ **Discitis and vertebral osteomyelitis in a patient after microdiscectomy.** Sagittal (A, B) and axial (C, D) T1-weighted images obtained before (left) and after (right) administration of gadolinium demonstrate destruction of the L3/4 intervertebral disc and collapse of adjacent vertebral bodies with hypointense marrow. There is contrast enhancement of the remaining intervertebral disc, adjacent vertebrae and paraspinal soft tissues.

are seen in the normal postoperative spine; a combination of imaging features (such as coexistence of intervertebral space enhancement, peridiscal signal changes and enhancing paraspinal mass) may be helpful.[3,14] Clinical correlation is crucial, and diagnosis may require percutaneous disc biopsy; this should be performed with a cutting needle, as aspiration leads to high proportion of false-negative results. The most serious form of postoperative infection requiring emergency surgical decompression or percutaneous drainage is spinal epidural abscess.[15] It can accompany spondylodiscitis or occur in isolation, and should be suspected when the patient demonstrates the triad of localised axial back pain, fever and progressive neurological deficit, ultimately leading to paraparesis. MRI demonstrates T1 hypointense, T2/STIR hyperintense epidural collection. The presence of contrast enhancement helps differentiate spinal epidural abscess from epidural haematoma, which otherwise can have similar appearances.

LATE COMPLICATIONS

Late complications of spinal surgery include delayed hardware failure and displacement leading to pseudoarthrosis and instability, as well as adjacent segment disease. A specific clinical entity termed 'failed back surgery syndrome' refers specifically to patients who have undergone lumbar spine surgery for degenerative disease (discectomy, foraminal stenosis or instability) and continue to experience symptoms due to a number of potential causes detailed below.

As mentioned earlier, hardware is used in spinal surgery to provide temporary support only and is destined to fail if the osseous fusion does not occur. In most cases hardware failure is, therefore, a manifestation of a lack of bony fusion and development of pseudoarthrosis. Factors that increase the risk of fusion failure include old age, smoking, diabetes, obesity, poor bone quality (e.g. in osteoporosis) and multilevel instrumentation. On plain radiographs pseudoarthrosis should be suspected if there is resorption of the bone graft, progressive misalignment, more than 4 mm translation or more than 10° of angular motion between adjacent vertebrae on flexion and extension views.[1,2] Features of pseudoarthrosis on cross-sectional imaging include a line between the bone and graft material that is lucent on CT, and a low T1 signal on MRI. Hardware failure such as fractured or extruded screws, fractured plates and rods and misplacement or subsistence of interbody cages can be evident on plain radiographs (Figs. 5-7A, B). CT allows more precise assessment of implants (Fig. 5-7C), and MRI may be helpful in evaluating compression of neural structures (Fig. 5-7D). On CT, the screws should be scrutinised for the presence of peri-implant lucency indicative of loosening; this is usually obvious in advanced cases (Fig. 5-7E), but early changes may be more subtle (Fig. 5-7F).

Adjacent segment disease is an accelerated occurrence of degenerative disc and facet changes at the level above and below the level of fusion due to altered spine dynamics. Imaging findings include typical degenerative changes

such as loss of disc height, disc herniation, endplate signal alterations and facet joint hypertrophy. The most important differential diagnosis is discitis and vertebral osteomyelitis, which, however, are likely to involve the site of surgery or fusion rather than the adjacent levels.

Failed Back Surgery Syndrome

Failed back surgery syndrome (FBSS) is a clinical entity defined as significant persistent back pain following surgical intervention with or without radiating pain and/or various degrees of functional incapacity.[16] Despite advances in technology and techniques, the number of patients suffering from FBSS has increased in recent years with increasing rate of spinal surgery.[17] The incidence of FBSS following lumbosacral spine surgery is reported to be between 10 and 40% in different studies.[9,18]

The aetiologies for FBSS can be classified in three main categories: preoperative, intraoperative and postoperative. The main preoperative risk factors are psychosocial influences, for example depression, anxiety or hypochondriasis.[19,20] Revision or repeated surgery is another preoperative risk factor, with the success rate decreasing to nearly half after second surgery and declining even further after subsequent operations.[21-23] Intraoperative causes of FBSS include poor technique, inadequate or overaggressive decompression and operation on the incorrect level. Overaggressive decompression may lead to spinal instability, which is seen in up to 14% of cases with FBSS. The incidence of incorrect operation level is widely variable in different studies, ranging from 0.03 to 3.3%,[24,25] and is increased in the presence of unusual patient characteristics such as morbid obesity, physical deformity or congenital variations. Emergency surgery, involvement of multiple surgeons or multiple procedures in a single surgical visit[26] and limited exposure in microscopic techniques[17] also increase the risk.

Postoperative causes for FBSS are those in which neuroimaging plays an important role. Residual or recurrent disc herniations are common following spinal surgery and can present with persistent or recurrent pain. Recurrent disease is seen in 7–12% cases of FBSS.[2] In the first few days after surgery it is difficult to differentiate the residual disc herniation from inflammatory tissue and debris. In the following weeks the inflammatory process and mass effect subside and avidly enhancing granulation tissue forms. After several months the granulation tissue reorganises to form epidural fibrosis, which demonstrates diffuse but weaker enhancement.[9] Differentiation between epidural scar and disc material is one of the most important and challenging aspects of postoperative spine imaging. Both disc material and epidural fibrosis are hypo- to isointense on T1-weighted and iso- to hyperintense on T2-weighted sequences, and gadolinium-enhanced T1-weighted images are crucial in their differentiation. Contrast-enhanced MRI has an accuracy of 96–100% for differentiating between fibrosis and disc material.[4] Recurrent or residual disc material does not enhance, or there is mild enhancement around the disc (Fig. 5-8). It is important to remember that contrast medium will penetrate the disc with time and the central part may show enhancement if imaging is delayed. It is

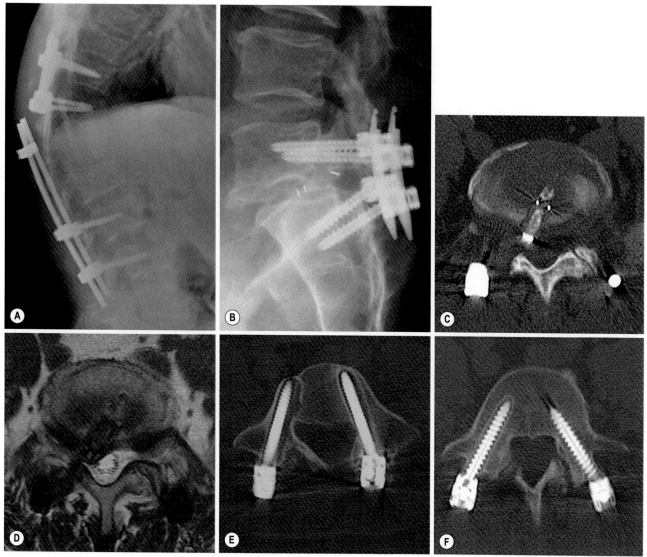

FIGURE 5-7 ■ **Examples of late hardware failure.** (A) Fractured rods in a patient with posterior thoracolumbar fixation of a burst fracture. (B) Posterior cage migration in a patient with transforaminal lumbar interbody fusion (TLIF); note that posterior radiopaque marker of the interbody cage lies within the spinal canal. (C) CT in the same patient allows better visualisation of the misplaced cage, and (D) axial T2-weighted MRI image demonstrates compression of the descending right S1 nerve root in the lateral recess by the misplaced cage. (E, F) Examples of various degree of peri-implant lucency indicating screws loosening; compare with normal left screw in (F).

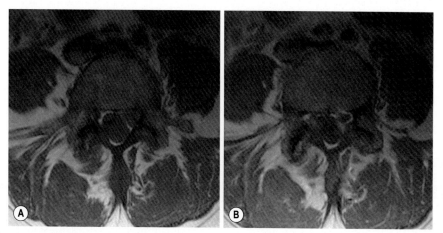

FIGURE 5-8 ■ **Example of a recurrent disc herniation.** (A) Unenhanced T1-weighted axial image demonstrates epidural lesion abutting the left anterior aspect of the thecal sac. (B) Gadolinium-enhanced image demonstrates peripheral enhancement, but the centre of the lesion remains of low signal.

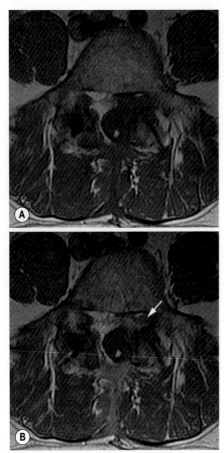

FIGURE 5-9 ■ Example of epidural fibrosis. (A) Unenhanced T1-weighted axial image demonstrates epidural lesion adjacent to the left anterior aspect of the theca. (B) Gadolinium-enhanced image demonstrates avid enhancement of the scar that extends along the left aspect of the thecal sac and is in continuity with postoperative scar tissue in the midline. Exiting nerve root (arrow) is surrounded by the enhancing tissue.

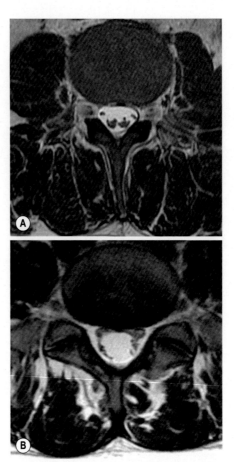

FIGURE 5-10 ■ Sterile arachnoiditis in patients following lumbar surgery. Axial T2-weighted images demonstrate clumping of nerve roots (A) and 'empty sac' sign (B) with nerve roots adherent to the periphery of the theca and absent in their usual dependent location.

therefore crucial that post-gadolinium images are obtained immediately after contrast injection. Herniated disc usually has smooth margins, lies anterolateral in the epidural space and tends to displace or compress the nerve roots and theca. On the other hand, epidural fibrotic tissue enhances early and uniformly, has irregular configuration with minimal mass effect and can occupy anterior-to-posterior aspects of the epidural space. It can also encase and retract the theca and nerve roots rather than displace them (Fig. 5-9). As epidural fibrosis is an inevitable finding following any surgery involving manipulation of the epidural space, it may be considered a normal postoperative change in the absence of significant theca deformity or tethering of nerve roots. Therefore, it is important to remember that symptoms may not be caused by the presence of epidural scar tissue, and that there is no correlation between severity of symptoms and the amount of scarring. Different studies have shown that epidural fibrosis can be responsible or contribute to pain in 20–36% of FBSS patients.[27,28] There are different theories regarding how epidural fibrosis causes persistent pain, including limitation of movement and

inflammation,[29] hypoxic damage to the nerve[30] or disturbance in CSF flow, resulting in nerve hypersensitivity.[31]

Sterile arachnoiditis is another postoperative cause of FBSS which has been reported in 6–16% of cases following spinal surgery.[4] The MRI features of arachnoiditis include 'clumping' of nerve roots and 'empty' theca caused by peripherally distributed nerve roots and their adhesion to the theca (Fig. 5-10), as well as an intrathecal soft-tissue 'mass' with a broad dural base representing a large group of matted nerve roots.

Nerve root enhancement on MRI is frequently seen in the early postoperative period, when it may reflect transient inflammation.[9] Enhancement present after 6 months should, however, be considered a pathological feature,[32] and suggests ongoing radiculitis as the cause of pain.[9] In asymptomatic patients nerve root enhancement is only rarely seen beyond this time point. In contrast, almost two-thirds of symptomatic patients demonstrate nerve root enhancement that strongly correlates with clinical symptoms, especially when combined with nerve thickening and displacement.[32]

Stenosis involving the central or juxta-articular portion of the spinal canal or neural foramen is an important cause of persistent or recurrent pain reported in 25 to

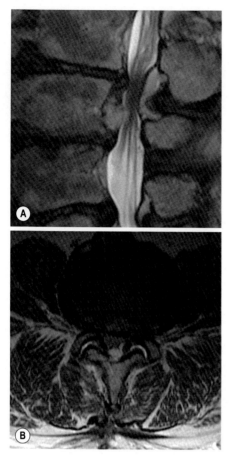

FIGURE 5-11 ■ Moderate spinal canal stenosis demonstrated on sagittal (A) and axial (B) T2-weighted images.

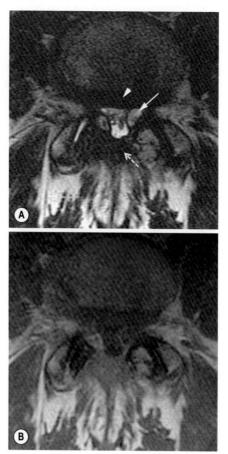

FIGURE 5-12 ■ Axial T2-weighted (A) and contrast-enhanced T1-weighted images (B) demonstrate a small synovial cyst (arrow) related to the left facet joint. Also note recurrent disc (arrowhead) and enhancing scar (dashed arrow) posteriorly. There is mild spinal canal stenosis.

29% of patients with FBSS.[33] Stenosis can be a consequence of accelerated degenerative changes after an operation. Loss of intervertebral disc height after discectomy is another cause. The best diagnostic clue on imaging is a trefoil appearance of the spinal canal on axial, and an hourglass appearance on sagittal imaging (Fig. 5-11). A sagittal diameter of the spinal canal less than 10 mm is considered absolute spinal canal stenosis.[2]

Postoperative synovial cysts (Fig. 5-12) are an uncommon cause of FBSS reported in 1% of cases. They are secondary to alteration of the facet joint biomechanics following surgery, with removal of ligamentum flavum as a potential predisposing factor. The important diagnostic clue is continuity of the cyst with the facet joint and the usual presence of fluid signal.[4]

IMAGE-GUIDED PERCUTANEOUS CEMENT BONE AUGMENTATION

Percutaneous cement bone augmentation interventions include vertebroplasty and kyphoplasty. The main indication for these procedures is pain associated with osteoporotic vertebral fractures refractory to medical therapy.[34,35] They may also be used in treatment of pathological vertebral fractures associated with lytic metastases

and multiple myeloma, as well as traumatic fractures. The treatment of asymptomatic vertebral compression fractures and prophylactic intervention in non-fractured vertebrae remain a matter of debate. It should be noted that effectiveness of vertebroplasty in relieving pain and improvement of function in patients with osteoporotic compression fractures has recently been in question in view of results of controlled randomised clinical trials showing no clinical benefit of the procedure,[36,37] or only modest reduction in pain with no difference in functional outcomes.[38] While the future role of cement bone augmentation remains to be established, differences between the techniques used and potential complications deserve a brief mention.

In vertebroplasty there is intraosseous injection of bone cement (usually PMMA; polymethylmethacrylate) into the vertebral body using a needle introduced via transpedicular approach under fluoroscopic guidance (Fig. 5-13A, B); extrapedicular or posterolateral approach can also be used. Partial restoration of vertebral height is sometimes accomplished, but is not a primary goal of the procedure. In kyphoplasty, before cement injection, inflatable tamps (balloons) are introduced into the vertebral body. Expanding tamps crush the trabeculae and create a cavity into which cement is instilled; some height

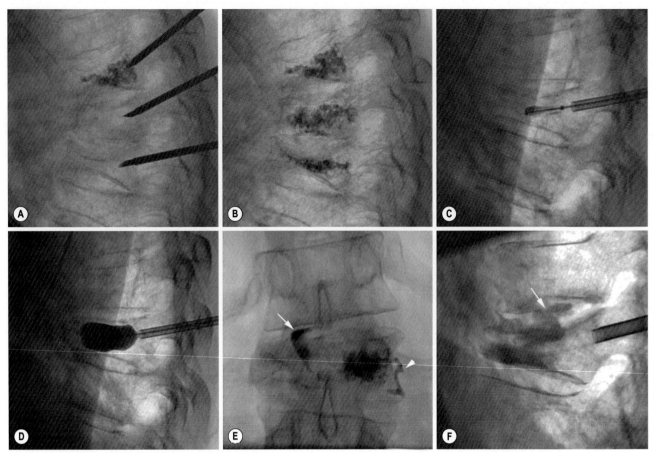

FIGURE 5-13 ■ **Fluoroscopic images obtained during cement bone augmentation procedures.** (A) Vertebroplasty on three adjacent levels showing transpedicular needles in situ and cement being injected at the most superior level. (B) Final effect of the vertebroplasty shown in (A). (C) Inflation of the balloon inside the vertebral body during kyphoplasty. Note partial reduction of the fracture (D) with some restoration of vertebral body height. (E, F) Extravasation of cement into the intervertebral space (arrows) increases risk of adjacent vertebral fracture post procedure. There is minor extravasation into a paravertebral vein (arrowhead in E).

restoration is more likely to be achieved (Figs. 5-13C, D). Variation of kyphoplasty aimed to maintain the degree of height restoration between the tamp deflation and cement injection involves deployment of balloon-mounted stents inside the vertebral body (stentoplasty).[39] The main potential complication of vertebroplasty is leakage of cement outside of the vertebral body, with extravasation into paravertebral veins (Fig. 5-13E); large extravasation with penetration of cement into systemic venous circulation may result in cement pulmonary emboli. Epidural or neural foraminal extravasation may lead to compression of neural structures requiring surgical decompression. Cement extravasation into the intervertebral space (Fig. 5-13F) has been shown to increase the risk of fractures of adjacent vertebrae post procedure.[35,40] Cement extravasation is less likely to happen in case of kyphoplasty thanks to lower viscosity of cement, which is instilled into a preformed cavity under lower pressure.[35] Other complications associated with needle placement include injury to epidural venous plexus, nerve roots or spinal cord.

REFERENCES

1. Benzel EC. Spine Surgery: Techniques, Complication Avoidance, and Management. 2nd ed. Philadelphia: Churchill Livingstone; 2005.
2. Ross JS. Specialty Imaging. Postoperative Spine. Philadelphia: Wolters Kluwer, Lippincott Williams & Wilkins; 2012.
3. Salgado R, Van Goethem JW, van den Hauwe L, Parizel PM. Imaging of the postoperative spine. Semin Roentgenol 2006;41:312–26.
4. Ginat TD, Murtagh R, Westesson P-eA. Imaging of postoperative spine. In: Atlas of Postsurgical Neuroradiology: Imaging of the Brain, Spine, Head, and Neck. 1st ed. Berlin: Springer; 2012.
5. Grabowski G, Cornett CA. Bone graft and bone graft substitutes in spine surgery: current concepts and controversies. J Am Acad Orthop Surg 2013;21:51–60.
6. Williams AL, Gornet MF, Burkus JK. CT evaluation of lumbar interbody fusion: current concepts. Am J Neuroradiol 2005;26:2057–66.
7. Mayer HM. Minimally Invasive Spine Surgery: A Surgical Manual. 2nd ed. London: Springer; 2005.
8. Douglas-Akinwande AC, Buckwalter KA, Rydberg J, et al. Multichannel CT: evaluating the spine in postoperative patients with orthopedic hardware. Radiographics 2006;26(Suppl 1):S97–110.
9. Van Goethem JW, Parizel PM, Jinkins JR. Review article: MRI of the postoperative lumbar spine. Neuroradiology 2002;44:723–39.
10. Mullin WJ, Heithoff KB, Gilbert TJ Jr, Renfrew DL. Magnetic resonance evaluation of recurrent disc herniation: is gadolinium necessary? Spine 2000;25:1493–9.
11. Stradiotti P, Curti A, Castellazzi G, Zerbi A. Metal-related artifacts in instrumented spine. Techniques for reducing artifacts in CT and MRI: state of the art. Eur Spine J 2009;18(Suppl 1):102–8.
12. Palumbo MA, Aidlen JP, Daniels AH, et al. Airway compromise due to wound hematoma following anterior cervical spine surgery. Open Orthop J 2012;6:108–13.

13. Aono H, Ohwada T, Hosono N, et al.. Incidence of postoperative symptomatic epidural hematoma in spinal decompression surgery. J Neurosurg Spine 2011;15:202–5.
14. Van Goethem JW, Parizel PM, van den Hauwe L, et al. The value of MRI in the diagnosis of postoperative spondylodiscitis. Neuroradiology 2000;42:580–5.
15. Grewal S, Hocking G, Wildsmith JA. Epidural abscesses. Br J Anaesth 2006;96:292–302.
16. Shafaie FF, Bundschuh C, Jinkins JR. The posttherapeutic lumbosacral spine. In: Jinkins JR, editor. Posttherapeutic Neurodiagnostic Imaging. Philadelphia: Lippincott-Raven; 1997.
17. Chan CW, Peng P. Failed back surgery syndrome. Pain Med 2011;12:577–606.
18. North RB, Campbell JN, James CS, et al. Failed back surgery syndrome: 5-year follow-up in 102 patients undergoing repeated operation. Neurosurgery 1991;28:685–90; discussion 690–1.
19. Celestin J, Edwards RR, Jamison RN. Pretreatment psychosocial variables as predictors of outcomes following lumbar surgery and spinal cord stimulation: a systematic review and literature synthesis. Pain Med 2009;10:639–53.
20. Mannion AF, Elfering A. Predictors of surgical outcome and their assessment. Eur Spine J 2006;15(Suppl 1):S93–108.
21. Fandino J, Botana C, Viladrich A, Gomez-Bueno J. Reoperation after lumbar disc surgery: results in 130 cases. Acta Neurochir (Wien) 1993;122:102–4.
22. Jonsson B, Stromqvist B. Repeat decompression of lumbar nerve roots. A prospective two-year evaluation. J Bone Joint Surg Br 1993;75:894–7.
23. Nachemson AL. Evaluation of results in lumbar spine surgery. Acta Orthop Scand Suppl 1993;251:130–3.
24. Mody MG, Nourbakhsh A, Stahl DL, et al. The prevalence of wrong level surgery among spine surgeons. Spine 2008;33:194–8.
25. Pao JL, Chen WC, Chen PQ. Clinical outcomes of microendoscopic decompressive laminotomy for degenerative lumbar spinal stenosis. Eur Spine J 2009;18:672–8.
26. Longo UG, Loppini M, Romeo G, et al. Errors of level in spinal surgery: an evidence-based systematic review. J Bone Joint Surg Br 2012;94:1546–50.
27. Fritsch EW, Heisel J, Rupp S. The failed back surgery syndrome: reasons, intraoperative findings, and long-term results: a report of 182 operative treatments. Spine 1996;21:626–33.
28. Ross JS, Robertson JT, Frederickson RC, et al. Association between peridural scar and recurrent radicular pain after lumbar discectomy: magnetic resonance evaluation. ADCON-L European Study Group. Neurosurgery 1996;38:855–61; discussion 861–3.
29. Robertson JT. Role of peridural fibrosis in the failed back: a review. Eur Spine J 1996;5(Suppl 1):S2–6.
30. Jayson MI. The role of vascular damage and fibrosis in the pathogenesis of nerve root damage. Clin Orthop Relat Res 1992;279:40–8.
31. Rydevik BL. The effects of compression on the physiology of nerve roots. J Manipulative Physiol Ther 1992;15:62–6.
32. Lee YS, Choi ES, Song CJ. Symptomatic nerve root changes on contrast-enhanced MR imaging after surgery for lumbar disk herniation. Am J Neuroradiol 2009;30:1062–7.
33. Waguespack A, Schofferman J, Slosar P, Reynolds J. Etiology of long-term failures of lumbar spine surgery. Pain Med 2002;3:18–22.
34. Bornemann R, Koch EM, Wollny M, Pflugmacher R. Treatment options for vertebral fractures an overview of different philosophies and techniques for vertebral augmentation. Eur J Orthop Surg Traumatol 2013;[Epub ahead of print].
35. Eck JC, Nachtigall D, Humphreys SC, Hodges SD. Comparison of vertebroplasty and balloon kyphoplasty for treatment of vertebral compression fractures: a meta-analysis of the literature. Spine J 2008;8:488–97.
36. Buchbinder R, Osborne RH, Ebeling PR, et al. A randomized trial of vertebroplasty for painful osteoporotic vertebral fractures. N Engl J Med 2009;361:557–68.
37. Kallmes DF, Comstock BA, Heagerty PJ, et al. A randomized trial of vertebroplasty for osteoporotic spinal fractures. N Engl J Med 2009;361:569–79.
38. Comstock BA, Sitlani CM, Jarvik JG, et al. Investigational Vertebroplasty Safety and Efficacy Trial (INVEST): patient-reported outcomes through 1 year. Radiology 2013;269(1):224–31.
39. Heini PF, Teuscher R. Vertebral body stenting/stentoplasty. Swiss Med Wkly 2012;142:w13658.
40. Nieuwenhuijse MJ, Putter H, van Erkel AR, Dijkstra PD. New vertebral fractures after percutaneous vertebroplasty for painful osteoporotic vertebral compression fractures: a clustered analysis and the relevance of intradiskal cement leakage. Radiology 2013;266:862–70.

SPINAL TRAUMA

James J. Rankine

CLINICAL ASPECTS

The cervical spine and thoracolumbar junction are the most common sites of spinal trauma. Specifically, the most common sites for fractures and dislocations are the lower cervical spine (C4–7), the thoracolumbar junction (T10–L2) and the craniocervical junction (C1–2). These mobile areas, particularly the cervical spine, can be injured with relatively little force. Patients with cervical trauma may present as 'walking wounded' to the accident and emergency departments with no other injuries and so despite the increasing use of CT as a first-line investigation, many patients with cervical trauma continue to be initially investigated with conventional radiographs. Approximately 15% of spinal fractures occur at more than one level and are non-contiguous, so the clinician must carefully assess the whole spine.[1]

In contrast to the cervical and lumbar spine, the thoracic spine is a relatively rigid structure, restricted in mobility by the thoracic cage. The thoracic spine, ribs and sternum constitute a bony ring and in common with fractures of bony rings elsewhere in the body, the ring often fractures at more than one point. A displaced fracture of the sternum should raise clinical suspicions of a fracture of the thoracic spine. Since greater forces are usually required to cause a thoracic spine fracture, associated vascular injury should be considered. For these reasons thoracic and lumbar trauma is most appropriately imaged as part of a polytrauma CT with intravenous contrast medium.

Patients with osteoporosis may sustain thoracic axial load compressive fractures with little or no history of injury and are often initially assessed by conventional radiographs. The lack of force involved in the injury should not imply to the clinician that these are fractures that always run a benign course. The compressed vertebral body can develop avascular necrosis, leading to delayed post-traumatic collapse and spinal deformity, termed Kummell's disease.[2] It is important that these patients are followed up clinically, and where appropriate their osteoporosis is pharmacologically treated.

Conventional radiographs cannot exclude injury in any part of the spine. While CT is sensitive to bony injury, it cannot exclude ligamentous disruption. This is particularly important in cervical trauma where the spine can be rendered unstable due to ligamentous disruption without any bony injury. The removal of spinal immobilisation in the light of negative conventional radiographs, or CT, should be performed in a controlled manner under senior supervision. Any clinical concerns, which are principally the degree of pain on gentle movement or the development of any neurological signs or symptoms, warrants an MRI examination, regardless of the findings on CT or conventional radiographs. It is important that the clinician managing a patient with spinal trauma is aware of the limitations of conventional radiographs and CT.

Patients with spinal injury should have regular neurological observations performed. Any clinical deterioration in the neurology warrants an urgent assessment by MRI to investigate the possibility of an epidural haematoma, which can be surgically drained. Urgent surgical intervention cannot correct any neurological dysfunction sustained at the time of injury, but can prevent worsening neurological damage from an expanding epidural haematoma compressing the spinal cord.

IMAGING TECHNIQUES AND EVALUATION

CERVICAL SPINE

Conventional Radiographs

A full conventional radiographic examination of the cervical spine as a minimum includes a lateral view, antero-posterior (AP) view and an AP odontoid peg view. The lateral view should include the cervical–thoracic junction, and if not then a 'swimmer's' view is performed where the arm adjacent to the radiographic plate is elevated and the beam is centred above the shoulder further from the plate and angled 15° in a cephalad direction. A full conventional radiographic examination is most appropriate in injury isolated to the cervical spine, with relatively low forces and where removal of immobilisation and clinical reassessment would be considered with negative findings. In many other situations, especially in the context of polytrauma, it is more appropriate to proceed directly to CT without conventional radiographs. Many institutions continue to perform a lateral radiograph as part of the initial assessment of the patient in the resuscitation room. Of the conventional radiographic projections, the lateral is the single most useful but with such rapid access to CT now available in most institutions the value of performing any conventional radiographs is debatable. The lateral radiograph no longer constitutes part of the primary survey in the ATLS guidelines[3] but cervical immobilisation must continue until the spine can be radiologically and clinically cleared.

Despite the diminishing role of conventional radiographs they remain a common means of initially assessing many patients and, since the principles of interpreting the radiographs also apply to the interpretation of the sagittal and coronal reformats produced by a CT examination, it remains an important skill.

Alignment is assessed by visually assessing the spinal lines on the lateral radiograph (Fig. 6-1). They should all appear smooth and without interruption. The anterior spinal line passes along anterior borders of the vertebral bodies and the anterior aspect of the odontoid peg. The distance between the anterior arch of C1 and the odontoid peg should not exceed 3 mm in adults and 5 mm in children. The posterior spinal line passes along the posterior borders of the vertebral bodies. The junction of the laminae with the spinous processes forms the spinolaminar line. The lamina of C2 is normally up to 2 mm posterior to the spinolaminar line. The facet joint line marks the posterior aspect of the facet joints and in a true lateral projection the facet joints on each side are superimposed, giving a single line. The distance between this line and the spinolaminar line should be the same at all levels. The appearance of a double facet joint line at a particular level is evidence of an abnormality of rotation at that level which is usually caused by a fracture disloca-tion of the facet joints (Fig. 6-2). The appearance of a double facet joint line is termed the 'bow tie' sign.

Slight anterior subluxation of C2 on C3 is a common normal appearance in children. In this situation the malalignment causes disruption of the anterior spinal line and

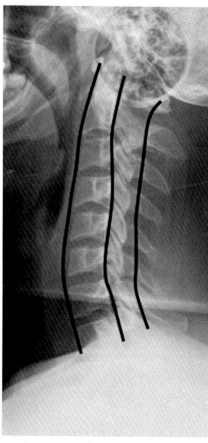

FIGURE 6-1 ■ Alignment on the lateral cervical spine radiograph is assessed by visually assessing the smooth contour of the spinal lines.

the spinolaminar line (Fig. 6-3). This distinguishes it from the Hangman's fracture, where the anterior spinal line is disrupted but the spinolaminar line is not, since the posterior elements are no longer connected to the vertebral body (see later).

Malalignment can occur with angulation of the spine in the absence of anterior subluxation. The distance between the spinous processes should be roughly equal at all levels, taking into account the normal downward slope of the C7 spinous process A kyphotic angulation of the spine associated with widening of the gap between two spinous processes implies rupture of the posterior ligamentous structures at that level (Fig. 6-4).

Noting the central position of the spinous processes assesses alignment on the AP radiograph. The spinous processes of the cervical spine may appear bifid (the spinous process separates into two portions). This is a normal anatomical finding at many levels and in this situation the central point of the posterior elements is the point midway between the two tubercles of the spinous process (which may be unequal in size).

When assessing the AP through mouth odontoid peg view, normal alignment is demonstrated by noting that the lateral margins of the C1–C2 facet joints are

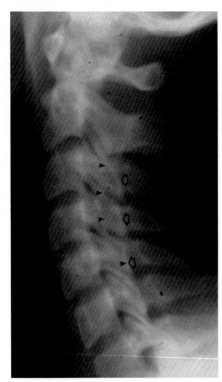

FIGURE 6-2 ■ **Unilateral facet joint dislocation.** The appearance of a double facet joint line, termed the bow tie sign (arrowheads and block arrows), on the lateral cervical radiograph is evidence of rotation of the spine.

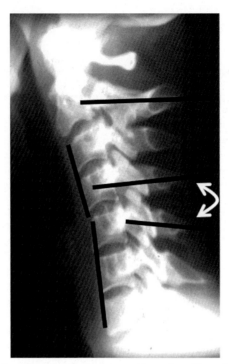

FIGURE 6-4 ■ **Posterior ligamentous disruption.** There is angulation of the anterior spinal line at C4–C5. The posterior lines mark the position of the spinous processes with fanning between the C4 and C5 spinous processes.

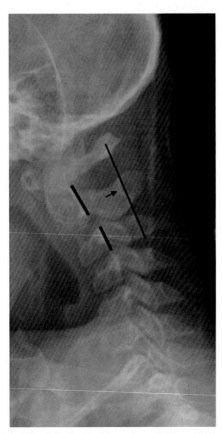

FIGURE 6-3 ■ **Physiological subluxation of C2 on C3 in a 6-year-old child.** There is disruption of the anterior and spinolaminar lines. The spinolaminar line of C2 (arrow) lies anterior to the spinolaminar line joining C1 and C3.

symmetrically aligned with no overlap. On the lateral view the integrity of Harris' ring should be examined at the base of the odontoid peg. This ring does not represent a distinct anatomical structure but is a composite shadow that includes the C2 body (Fig. 6-5).

The bones are assessed for fractures, cortical disruption and separate bony fragments. A well-corticated round opacity situated at the site of the anterior longitudinal ligament should not be mistaken for an avulsion. The lack of cortical disruption of the adjacent vertebral body and the absence of soft-tissue swelling are indicators of this normal finding, which is thought to represent a remnant of an ununited secondary vertebral ossification centre.

Soft-tissue swelling is assessed on the lateral radiograph. Superior to the level of the larynx the distance between the anterior aspect of the vertebral bodies and the posterior aspect of the air in the oropharynx should be no greater than one-third of the AP diameter of a vertebral body width. Inferior to the level of the larynx (usually C3 or C4 and frequently seen due to calcification in the laryngeal cartilage) it should be no greater than the AP diameter of the vertebral body. Intubation distorts the soft tissues behind the oropharynx, making the interpretation of soft-tissue swelling unreliable in intubated patients.

Lateral flexion and extension radiographs have traditionally been used to assess stability of the spine. Movement of the acutely injured spine in the presence of ligamentous disruption can cause neurological injury so there is no role for flexion and extension radiographs in the acutely injured spine. The stability of the spine and the presence of ligamentous disruption should be assessed by MRI. There remains a role for flexion and extension radiographs in the assessment of delayed instability, but this is likely to be some months after the acute event and should only take place after appropriate imaging and treatment of the acutely injured spine.

CT

CT of the cervical spine should include the spine from the cranio-cervical junction to the level of the third thoracic vertebral body. The precise imaging parameters will depend on the CT system being used, but an appropriately thin slice thickness should be selected to allow good-quality coronal and sagittal reformats. The alignment and soft-tissue swelling is assessed on these reformats using the same basic principles as the interpretation of the conventional radiograph. The axial sections are particularly useful for diagnosing bone fractures.

The presence of malalignment and soft-tissue swelling will often give an indication of ligamentous disruption in the absence of any bony injury but this is not always the case. If there is continued clinical concern following a normal CT, then MRI is warranted as CT cannot exclude a purely ligamentous disruption.

MRI

MRI of the cervical spine is best performed with the standard head and neck coils for the particular system being used to allow the best resolution with a small field of view. As there are frequently fractures at multiple levels the whole of the spine should be imaged in the sagittal plane. Axial sections can be planned from the sagittal slices and targeted at areas of abnormality. The principles of the sequences used and the image interpretation apply equally to the cervical spine and thoracolumbar spine.

The sagittal sequences should include T1- and T2-weighted fat-saturated sequences. A short tau inversion recovery (STIR) sequence can be used as an alternative to the T2-weighted fat-saturated sequence since it is a robust sequence that provides reliable fat suppression. Bone and soft-tissue injury is more clearly demonstrated with fat-saturated sequences and injuries can be missed on standard turbo spin echo T2-weighted sequences (Fig. 6-6).

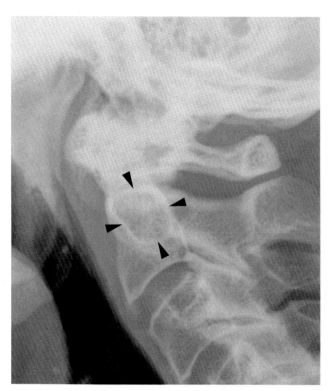

FIGURE 6-5 ■ Harris' ring. The normal lateral cervical spine film shows an an apparent ring at the base of the odontoid peg (arrowheads). This does not correspond to a single anatomical structure but is a composite shadow which includes the C2 vertebral body.

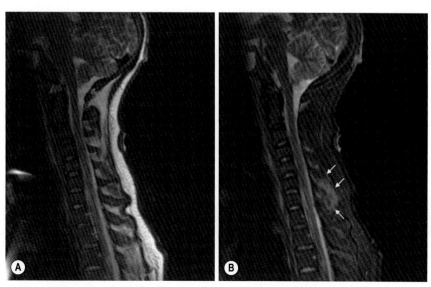

FIGURE 6-6 ■ (A) Sagittal T2-weighted and (B) STIR MRI. There is a fracture of the posterior elements of C5, which is demonstrated by oedematous change on the STIR sequence (arrows) but not seen on the T2-weighted sequence.

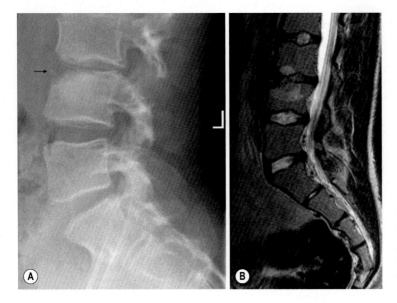

FIGURE 6-7 ■ **Limbus vertebrae.** (A) Conventional radiograph and (B) sagittal T2-weighted fat-saturated MRI in a 14-year-old male. The antero-superior endplate of L4 is depressed with a separate bone fragment (arrow). The MRI demonstrates that the intervertebral disc has prolapsed anteriorly, separating the bone fragment from the vertebral body. There is associated bone oedema, indicating this is a relatively recent occurrence.

Gradient echo sequences may be used when assessing neurological injury since these better demonstrate haemorrhage, an important prognostic indicator for poor neurological recovery.

THORACOLUMBAR SPINE

Conventional Radiographs

The conventional radiographic examination of the thoracic and lumbar spine includes AP and lateral views. The upper thoracic spine is particularly difficult to image on the lateral view due to the substantial overlying bone and soft tissues of the shoulders. CT, as part of a polytrauma CT protocol, most appropriately images the thoracic spine, as greater forces are required to cause a fracture of the relatively rigid thoracic cage. Conventional radiographs of the thoracic spine are rightly becoming a rare investigation.

Soft-tissue swelling due to a paravertebral haematoma is best demonstrated on the AP view of the thoracic spine where it causes focal widening of the mediastinum. Alignment is assessed on both the AP and lateral views. There should be an equal distance between the spinous processes and on the AP view the spinous process should be central with a symmetrical appearance of the pedicles and vertebral body.

The greater degree of mobility of the spine at the thoracolumbar junction renders this area particularly prone to injury and it is a relatively easy area to demonstrate with conventional radiographs due to the even quantity of overlying soft tissue. Patients with osteoporosis can sustain vertebral body compression fractures with fairly minimal forces. Often the challenge in interpreting the conventional radiograph is in determining what is an acute injury and what is old. Acute fractures tend to have sharp cortical margins and lucent fracture lines, whereas old injuries have smooth cortical margins and sclerosis.

Ultimately, clinical correlation and, if necessary, MRI are a more reliable indicator of the age of a fracture than conventional radiographs.

A limbus vertebrae is a common developmental abnormality that should not be confused with an acute injury (Fig. 6-7). In the lumbar spine it most commonly affects the superior endplate of L4. These usually occur during adolescence before the endplates develop their full structural integrity. The intervertebral disc can prolapse anteriorly, lifting off the ring apophysis, typically occurring without any history of injury. The typical site and well-corticated appearance of the bone fragment are clues that this is not an acute injury.

CT

CT of the thoracic and lumbar spine should be performed as part of a polytrauma CT protocol that includes an intravenous contrast agent for the assessment of vascular injury. The precise imaging parameters will depend on the particular CT system but the axial imaging should allow sagittal and coronal reformats of sufficient diagnostic quality. The sagittal reformats of the thoracic spine should include the sternum since this is part of the bony ring of the thoracic cage and the integrity of the sternum is important in the stability of a thoracic fracture.

Because of the relatively rigid nature of the thoracic spine, injury usually involves bony fractures. CT is therefore very useful for diagnosing or excluding a thoracic spine injury. The thoracolumbar junction, on the other hand, is a relatively mobile structure and behaves more like the cervical spine in that purely ligamentous injury can occur without bony fractures. The presence of epidural fat within the spinal canal adjacent to the ligamentum flavum provides a natural soft-tissue contrast for assessing the posterior ligaments, an anatomical feature which is not present in the cervical spine (see later). However, ultimately, MRI remains the gold standard for assessing purely ligamentous injury.

SPECIFIC INJURY PATTERNS

CERVICAL SPINE

Atlanto-Occipital Dissociation

Dissociation between the cranium and cervical spine is an unusual injury since it is usually incompatible with life. It more commonly occurs in children. A simple assessment of normal cranial–cervical alignment is provided by tracing a line down the clivus that should extend onto the tip of the odontoid process. With cranio-cervical dislocation this line will fall anterior or posterior to the tip of the odontoid peg (Fig. 6-8).

C1 Injuries

Rotatory Subluxation

Fixed rotatory subluxation occurs most frequently in children and typically occurs following a respiratory illness in the absence of trauma. The hallmark feature is fixed rotation between C1 and C2. An inadequately positioned CT performed with the head rotated to one side can mimic a rotatory subluxation since the function of the C1–C2 joint is to allow rotation of the head relative to the spine. Re-positioning the head and reimaging will correct the rotation, whereas in fixed rotatory subluxation the rotation between C1 and C2 persists when the patient rotates the head to either side. With this pattern of malalignment there is usually no history of trauma and when diagnosed in the context of acute trauma it is most frequently a case of misdiagnosis due to inadequate positioning at the time of CT rather than true rotatory subluxation and the first step should be to review the positioning of the patient and if necessary repeat the examination.

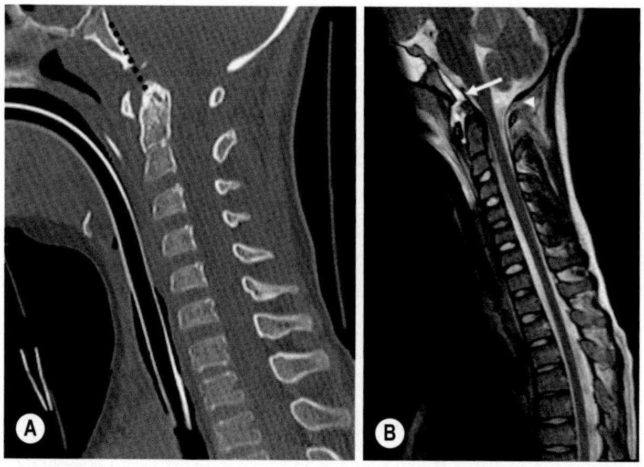

Jefferson Fracture

Fractures of the C1 ring, in common with fractures of bony rings elsewhere in the body, usually fracture at more than one site. A Jefferson fracture describes a fracture involving the anterior and posterior ring due to an axial force transmitted through the occipital condyles onto the atlas. The disruption of the anterior and posterior ring results in malalignment of the C1–C2 facet joints. The diagnosis can be made on conventional radiograph open mouth peg views, where overhanging of the lateral mass of C1 will be seen relative to the margins of C2 (Fig. 6-9A). However, CT will best demonstrate the site and any associated soft-tissue mass (Fig. 6-9B). On the open mouth peg view, simple asymmetry of the spaces between the odontoid peg and lateral masses is not diagnostic of this fracture pattern. Incomplete ossification of the posterior arch of C1 is a common normal variant that should not be confused with a fracture.

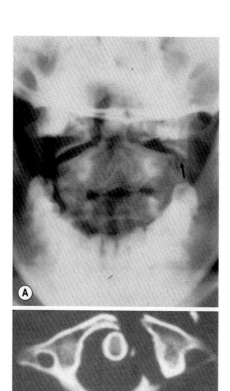

FIGURE 6-8 ■ **Atlanto-occipital dissociation.** (A) A line drawn down the clivus passes onto the anterior aspect of the odontoid peg (dashed line). (B) Sagittal STIR sequence. The apical ligament (arrow), which is the superior extension of the posterior longitudinal ligament, is stripped off the clivus. The cranium is anteriorly subluxed relative to the cervical spine. There is oedema (arrowhead) related to the posterior ligamentous disruption.

FIGURE 6-9 ■ **Jefferson fracture.** (A) Open mouth odontoid peg view. There is overhanging of the C1–C2 facet joint on the left (arrow)—compare with the right. (B) Axial CT demonstrates anterior and posterior ring fractures.

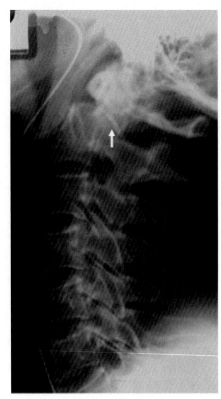

FIGURE 6-10 ■ **Fracture of the base of the odontoid peg with posterior displacement (arrow).** The anterior spinal line runs up the anterior aspect of the arch of C1 and not the odontoid peg.

C2 Injuries

Odontoid Fractures

Fracture of the odontoid peg is a relatively common injury. The classic diagnostic feature is displacement of the anterior C1 arch relative to C2 (Fig. 6-10). Displacement is usually posterior though the fracture can displace anteriorly. With an undisplaced fracture the only diagnostic clue may be soft-tissue swelling anterior to the upper cervical spine.

The fracture either occurs through the base of the odontoid peg (type II fracture) or extends into the body of C2 (type III). A type III fracture has a better prognosis for bony union since there is a greater vascular supply in the vertebral body than in the peg. The diagnosis of an undisplaced type III fracture can be difficult but is aided by examining Harris' ring (see Fig. 6-5).[4] A type III fracture extends into the body of C2 and can be seen as a disruption of the ring (Fig. 6-11).

A type I fracture describes an avulsion of the tip of the odontoid peg, a controversial condition that is never encountered in clinical practice in acute trauma. An os odontoideum is a well-corticated ossification centre above a rudimentary peg which is not a feature of acute injury though some consider it the sequela of a type I injury.

Hangman's Fracture

A hangman's fracture is a traumatic spondylolisthesis of C2 where a fracture occurs through both pedicles,

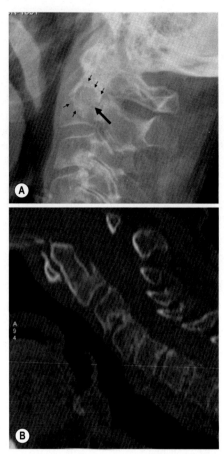

FIGURE 6-11 ■ **Undisplaced type III odontoid peg fracture.** (A) Harris' ring (arrows) is disrupted posteriorly (large arrow)—compare with Fig. 6-5. (B) CT Sagittal reformat showing the fracture is minimally displaced.

separating the posterior elements from the vertebral body (Fig. 6-12). The C2 vertebral body subluxes anteriorly relative to C3 but the posterior elements remain normally aligned. Because the spinal canal effectively widens in AP diameter at the level of slip there is often little or no neurological injury despite sometimes marked spondylolisthesis.

Hyperflexion Injuries

Flexion forces to the spine can cause rupture of the posterior elements, resulting in kyphotic angulation and anterior displacement. Typically there may be little in the way of anterior soft-tissue swelling since all the soft-tissue injury occurs posteriorly. If no associated bony injury occurs, then the diagnosis rests on demonstrating the abnormality of alignment (see Fig. 6-4).

There may be a fracture of the anterior aspect of the vertebral body, the flexion teardrop fracture. The bony fragment is typically relatively large and elongated in the cranio-caudal direction of the spine, which distinguishes it from the hyperextension tear drop, which is usually a small fragment. Since significant spinal displacement is required at the time of injury to cause such a compression fracture there is a strong association with severe neurological injury.

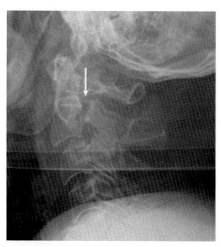

FIGURE 6-12 ■ Hangman's fracture. There is a fracture between the pedicles and body of C2 (arrow). There is slight anterior subluxation of C2 on C3 but the spinolaminar line of C2 remains behind the spinolaminar line of C1 and C3 (compare with physiological subluxation depicted in Fig. 6-3).

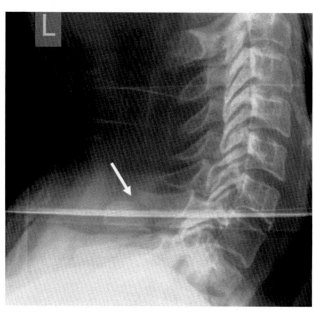

FIGURE 6-14 ■ Clay-shoveler's fracture. There is a fracture of the spinous process of C7 (arrow), which does not extend to the spinolaminar line.

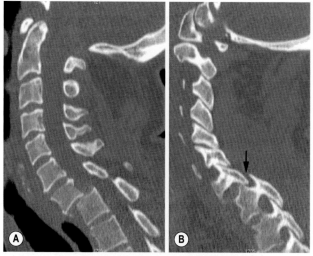

FIGURE 6-13 ■ Bilateral facet joint dislocation. (A) Sagittal CT reformat. There is greater than 50% forward slip of C7 on T1. (B) Parasagittal reformat through the facet joint demonstrates that the joints are 'locked' in a dislocated position (arrow).

Bilateral subuxation of the facet joints can occur with little in the way of bony injury. The facet joints can lock in a displaced position, the so-called perched facet joints (Fig. 6-13). The displacement of the spine can be 50% or greater of the vertebral body width.

A hyperflexion force with resistance of the posterior paraspinal muscles can produce a 'clay-shoveler's' fracture (Fig. 6-14). This is a fracture of the lower cervical or upper thoracic spinous process and is one of the few cervical fractures that can be considered stable. The fracture should not extend across the spinolaminar line as this suggests injury to the posterior ligaments and hence instability.

Hyperflexion Rotation Injury

A rotational force applied along with flexion can result in a unilateral dislocation of a facet joint. The key conventional radiographic feature is the demonstration of a rotational abnormality at a single level (see Fig. 6-2). Malalignment in the sagittal plane may be very minimal so the abnormality of rotation is a key diagnostic feature. CT demonstrates the 'reverse hamburger' sign on the axial sections through the facet dislocation (Fig. 6-15). The use of CT in this injury has demonstrated that a dislocation of the facet joint is frequently associated with a fracture of the joint and that these are not usually purely ligamentous injuries as previously thought.

Hyperextension Injuries

Extension force to the spine can result in rupture of the anterior longitudinal ligament and posterior displacement and angulation. There is typically soft-tissue swelling anterior to the spine at the site of the ligamentous disruption and since the malalignment may be very subtle the presence of this soft-tissue swelling is a key sign. There may be an associated hyperextension teardrop fracture, which is usually a small fragment (Fig. 6-16).

Neurological abnormality implies that a hyperextension dislocation occurred at the time of injury though the spine may be relatively normally aligned subsequently. This is the usual mechanism of injury when a patient has clinical signs of neurological damage in the presence of relatively normal conventional radiographs and CT imaging. The term *spinal cord injuries without radiological abnormality* (SCIWORA) has been applied in the past to this situation, a condition more commonly seen in children. However, any patient with neurological abnormality following acute trauma warrants an MRI which

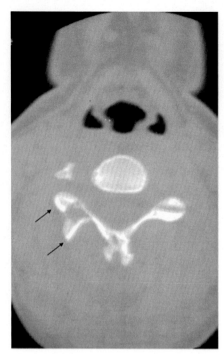

FIGURE 6-15 ■ **Unilateral facet joint dislocation.** The left facet joint has a 'hamburger' appearance. The right facet joint is dislocated and fractured, giving the appearances of the 'reverse hamburger' sign (arrows).

will demonstrate the soft-tissue injuries, so the term SCIWORA is probably an anachronism.

THORACIC AND LUMBAR SPINE

Classification Systems

Classifying a spinal fracture provides an important tool for the radiologist in communicating with the treating surgeon. For the surgeon it provides a guide to the management, the most crucial decision being the need for surgical internal fixation versus conservative treatment. Ideally a classification system would identify those injuries which are unstable: that is liable to continuing deformity or neurological injury under normal physiological loads. Denis described a three-column concept of the spine, the middle column involving the posterior aspect of the vertebral body and posterior longitudinal ligament, the anterior column the structures anterior to this and the posterior column the structures posterior.[5] Traditional teaching has been that any injury that involves two of the three columns is unstable but this is a gross simplification. One of the commonest thoracic and lumbar injuries is the burst fracture that according to Denis' concept involves the anterior and middle columns and is therefore unstable, yet many burst fractures are stable and treated non-operatively. Conversely, apparently minor endplate fractures in the presence of osteoporosis can progress to avascular necrosis and delayed vertebral collapse and deformity. The purely anatomical disruption of the spine is only one factor in determining the management of the patient, but it is important for the

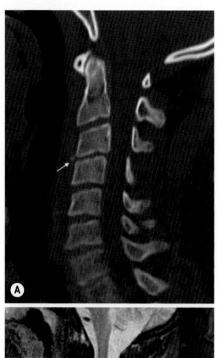

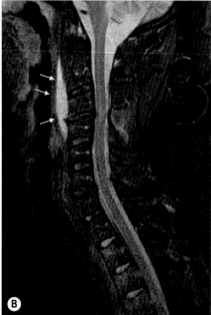

FIGURE 6-16 ■ **Hyperextension injury.** (A) Sagittal CT reformat. There is a small hyperextension teardrop fracture (arrow). There is slight malalignment at C3–C4 with retrolisthesis. (B) Sagittal STIR MRI. There is a large amount of anterior soft-tissue swelling (arrows). There is evidence of cord injury with cord oedema.

radiologist to accurately identify the extent of the bony and ligamentous disruption.

More recent classification systems have been described to take into account the anatomical information available on MRI. Oner et al.[6] described a classification system that categorised all the possible relevant structures seen on MRI, which included the endplate, the disc and the ligamentous structures. The AO classification system[7] provides a comprehensive system for describing the mechanism and anatomical disruption of the spine. The problem for the reporting radiologist in these systems lies in their complexity: the AO system has 22 different categories.

The system described in this chapter is necessarily simplistic and based on the Denis classification that has a mechanistic and anatomical approach. The importance in pattern recognition is in identifying those situations in which the degree of ligamentous disruption is likely to be greater than initially apparent on conventional radiographs or CT. MRI can then be performed in these cases, allowing a more accurate description of the anatomical disruption.

Flexion Compression and Flexion Distraction Injuries

The flexion compression fracture results in loss of height of the anterior aspect of the vertebral body but the posterior ligamentous structures are intact. The flexion distraction injury ruptures the posterior bony and/or ligamentous structures by distraction and causes a variable degree of compression of the anterior column (Fig. 6-17). The posterior ligamentous structures that are ruptured include the posterior longitudinal ligament, the ligamentum flavum, the interspinous ligament and the supraspinous ligament. Often the posterior distraction will occur through the posterior bony elements, the so-called bony Chance fracture, named after the British radiologist who first described the injury.[8] These are relatively easy to identify since the bony injury can be seen on conventional radiographs and is easily

demonstrable by CT. The fracture may occur through one vertebra, passing through the pedicles and spinous process at a single level. In this pure bony Chance fracture the posterior ligaments remain intact and while these fractures are usually surgically fixed there is a good prognosis since bony injury heals better than ligamentous disruption. The fracture may pass through the pars interarticularis and involve the posterior ligaments of the adjacent level, usually the level above. This is an important observation since it will determine the extent of surgical fixation. With the advent of CT multislice technology, allowing reformats of high quality, it is becoming apparent that CT can define the posterior ligamentous structures. The presence of epidural fat adjacent to the ligamentum flavum provides a natural anatomical contrast to the density of the ligament. The intact ligament should have a smooth contour, whereas irregularity implies a rupture. With rupture of the ligament, haemorrhage occurs into the epidural fat, giving a 'dirty fat' sign (Fig. 6-18). However, ultimately, MRI remains the most accurate means of demonstrating ligamentous disruption

If the flexion distraction injury involves the posterior ligamentous structures without posterior bony injury this is referred to as a soft-tissue Chance injury (Fig. 6-17B). Without bony injury present these can provide a diagnostic challenge on conventional radiographs and CT, as they can be confused with the simple flexion compression

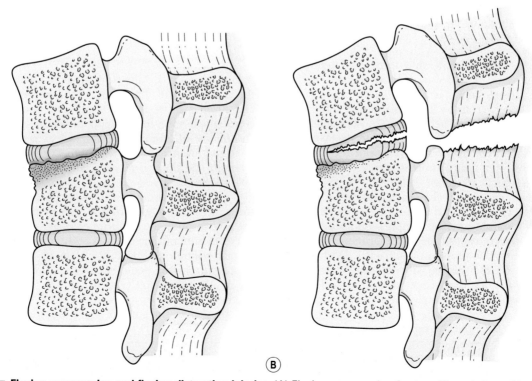

FIGURE 6-17 ■ **Flexion compression and flexion distraction injuries.** (A) Flexion compression fracture. There is loss of height of the anterior aspect of the vertebral body. The posterior ligaments are intact. (B) Flexion distraction injury. There is rupture of the posterior ligaments and only slight compression of the anterior vertebral body. The illustration shows disruption at the level of the intervertebral disc without posterior bony fracture, a 'soft-tissue Chance' injury. However, the fracture may pass through the bone elements of the posterior arch (bony Chance fracture).

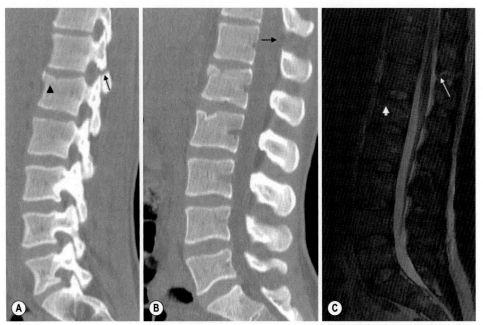

FIGURE 6-18 ■ Flexion distraction injury with bony and ligamentous involvement. (A) There is anterior compression of the vertebral body (arrowhead) and a fracture through the pars interarticularis (arrow). (B) The distraction injury extends through the interspinous ligament of the level above. There is a 'dirty fat' sign with loss of the normal epidural fat (arrow). (C) Sagittal T2-weighted MRI; there is compression of the anterior aspect of the vertebral body (arrowhead) and interspinous ligament disruption of the level above (arrow) with disruption of the ligamentum flavum and high signal passing through the interspinous ligament.

injury with intact posterior ligaments. The diagnostic clues begin before the imaging, with the degree of clinical suspicion relating to the mechanism of injury. Elderly patients with osteoporosis can sustain compression fractures of the vertebral body with minimal force, whereas it usually requires considerable force to fracture the young adult spine. The degree of bony compression in a soft-tissue Chance injury is usually fairly minimal since the flexion occurs around a fulcrum anterior to the spine: for instance, in a lap seat belt injury. Considerable vertebral body collapse is more suggestive of an axial compressive injury and if this involves the posterior vertebral wall then the posterior ligamentous structures will be intact since this is a burst fracture (see later).

The main diagnostic clue to a soft-tissue Chance injury is a kyphotic spinal deformity. A kyphosis can occur with a simple anterior compression injury but the degree of deformity will be commensurate with the degree of bony compression (Fig. 6-19). With a soft-tissue Chance, the degree of deformity cannot be explained by the degree of vertebral compression, which is usually slight. Unfortunately the demonstration of a kyphotic deformity is variable and depends on the positioning of the patient at the time of imaging (Fig. 6-20). The lack of a kyphotic deformity cannot therefore be used as evidence of intact posterior ligaments.

In addition to carefully reviewing the lateral films for evidence of a suspected Chance injury, evidence of bone or soft-tissue injury to the posterior elements may be evident on the AP film, which should also be carefully reviewed. Fracture through the pedicles or spinous processes and/or widening of the gap between adjacent spinous processes (which should normally be equidistant) are important features of Chance injuries (Fig. 6-21).

Burst Fractures

A burst fracture results from an axial compressive force through the spine. This is one of the commonest thoracic and lumbar spine fractures and can also occur in the cervical spine if a force is applied to the top of the head without significant neck flexion or extension. In the thoracic and lumbar spine a typical mechanism is a fall from a height and there is an association with bilateral calcaneal fractures.

The vertebral body, pedicles and posterior bony structures constitute a bony ring so that there is commonly a fracture through the posterior elements in addition to the burst fracture of the vertebral body. This combination of a body fracture and posterior element fracture can lead to splaying of the pedicles, a feature which can be seen on an AP radiograph (Fig. 6-22). The hallmark feature on the lateral projection is loss of vertebral body height, which involves the anterior and posterior vertebral body walls. This loss of height of the posterior vertebral wall distinguishes this injury from a flexion compression and flexion distraction injury in which the posterior wall is intact. Compression of the posterior vertebral wall in the context of other typical features of a burst fracture effectively excludes disruption of the posterior ligaments since the posterior structures have been compressed and not distracted (Fig. 6-23).

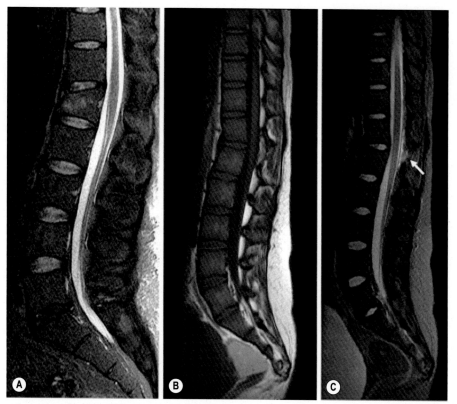

FIGURE 6-19 ■ **Comparing the kyphosis in flexion compression and flexion distraction injuries.** (A) Flexion compression injury, sagittal STIR MRI. There is a moderate degree of anterior compression of the vertebral body but only minimal kyphosis. The posterior ligaments are intact. (B) Sagittal T1-weighted and (C) sagittal STIR MRI. Flexion distraction, soft-tissue Chance injury. Kyphosis in the absence of any vertebral body compression. There is disruption of the posterior ligaments (arrow).

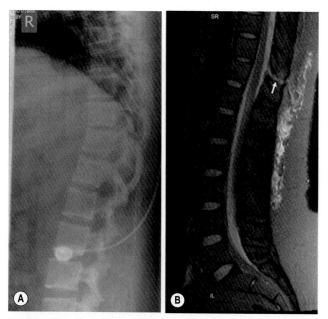

FIGURE 6-20 ■ **Soft-tissue Chance injury.** (A) Lateral radiograph shows a kyphotic deformity. (B) Same patient, sagittal STIR MRI. With the patient lying supine in the MRI unit there is no spinal deformity despite an interspinous ligament disruption (arrow).

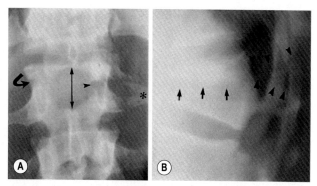

FIGURE 6-21 ■ **Bony Chance fracture of L1.** The AP projection (A) shows a comminuted fracture of the left transverse process (*), transverse fracture of the left pedicle (arrowhead), separation of the T12 and L1 spinous processes (double arrow) and a fracture of the right superolateral cortex of L1 (curved arrow). In the lateral projection (B) the arrowheads indicate a distraction transverse fracture of the spinous process and laminae and the arrows indicate the horizontal fracture of the body with anterior wedging.

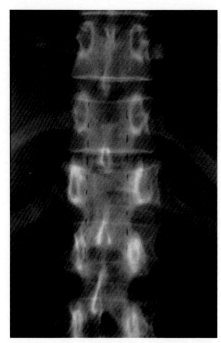

FIGURE 6-22 ■ **AP radiograph of a burst fracture.** The pedicle of the fractured vertebra lies outside a line joining the inner aspects of the pedicles of the level above and below (dotted line).

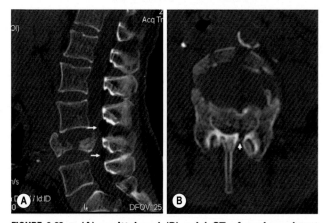

FIGURE 6-23 ■ **(A) sagittal and (B) axial CT of a pincer burst fracture.** There is loss of height of the vertebral body affecting the anterior and posterior walls. The presence of normal epidural fat (absence of the 'dirty fat' sign)(arrows) is evidence of intact ligaments. Note the ligamentum flavum buckles into the spinal canal. There is a fracture of the lamina (arrowhead).

There may be a mild kyphotic deformity if the anterior vertebral body collapses more than the posterior wall. A fragment from the anterior vertebral body wall may separate, resulting in a 'pincer burst' fracture. A progressive kyphotic deformity can develop in this situation if the fragment fails to unite with the rest of the vertebral body. For this reason pincer fractures are usually surgically fixed.

Lateral asymmetrical collapse of the vertebral body may lead to a lateral plane deformity (lateral angulation or curvature) evident on the AP projection and CT coronal reformats. Whilst there is frequently a degree of angulation deformity at the fracture site there is no step

in the alignment without a spondylolisthesis on the lateral or sagittal projections and no lateral step on the AP or coronal views. This distinguishes a burst fracture from a fracture dislocation, which may have fractures of the anterior and posterior vertebral body walls but also has complete ligamentous disruption including all the posterior ligaments, a highly unstable injury.

The axial CT section through a burst fracture shows the typical appearance of encroachment of the posterior vertebral wall into the spinal canal and burst fractures are strongly associated with neurological injury (Fig. 6-23B). Wilcox et al. performed high-speed video filming and pressure monitoring at the moment of burst fracture in an animal model.[9] They demonstrated that all the neurological injury occurs at the moment of the burst fracture and the resting state of the fragment in the canal has no bearing on subsequent neurological injury. This resting position of the fragment is the appearance demonstrated on CT and, whilst the size of the fragment in the canal may seem alarming, surgeons no longer routinely surgically remove these fragments, given it has no bearing on the neurological outcome.[10] If, following neurological improvement, the patient subsequently develops signs of canal stenosis, this can be addressed later, after the acute event.

The CT appearances of a burst fracture are so characteristic that the role of MRI is principally in demonstrating the associated neurological injury. Since there is frequently a fracture of the bony posterior elements, oedematous change will frequently be seen in the interspinous ligament adjacent to the fractured lamina. This should not be confused with a rupture of the ligament. The ligamentum flavum frequently appears buckled, a result of loss of height of the vertebral body, but no defect will be seen in the ligament.

Fracture Dislocation

A combination of flexion and rotation can result in a fracture dislocation in the thoracic and lumbar spine. These are high force injuries, which are frequently associated with severe neurological injury and often cord transection. There will be varying degrees of bony disruption, but the full width of the spine is always involved, with complete ligamentous disruption, making these the most unstable of injuries.

The key diagnostic feature is a step in the alignment in either the sagittal or coronal profile, frequently both (Fig. 6-24). Any step in alignment within the thoracic spine implies a fracture dislocation since a step in alignment is not encountered in other conditions. In the lumbar spine a spondylolisthesis is frequently encountered due to degenerative disease at L4–L5 and spondylolysis at L5–S1. A step in the lateral plane can be seen in association with a degenerative lumbar scoliosis but these conditions have typical features and, in the absence of other features of injury, should not cause any diagnostic confusion.

An MRI should always be performed in these injuries to investigate the neurological injury and as a preoperative plan. Fragments of bone, disc or haematoma within the canal can worsen the neurological injury if realignment of the spine causes these to exert a greater pressure effect on the cord. In the case of cord transection with complete neurological paralysis, this will not be a consideration although the spine is frequently still surgically stabilised to aid the patient's rehabilitation.

THE RIGID SPINE

The patient presenting with a fracture through an otherwise fused spine presents specific problems in their diagnosis and management. The commonest causes of spinal fusion are ankylosing spondylitis (AS) and diffuse idiopathic skeletal hyperostosis (DISH). The lack of a motion segment in the fused spine gives it the biomechanical properties of a long bone. When a fracture occurs through the fused spine it always occurs through the full width of the spine and is highly unstable. The presence of osteoporosis in a fused spine, coupled with the biomechanical properties of an extended lever arm, can result in a fracture with a minimal history of trauma. The clinician must be aware of the possibility of a highly unstable fracture in a patient with new onset of symptoms in the fused spine, even in the absence of any history of trauma. In treating these fractures extensive surgical fixation is required to overcome the biomechanics of an extended lever arm, similar to the principles of long bone fixation.

The fracture through the fused spine usually runs in the transverse plane. If the fracture is undisplaced and the bones are osteoporotic the fracture line may be very indistinct and require high-quality coronal and sagittal CT imaging. The presence of gas within the fused spine is an indicator of motion and hence fracture (Fig. 6-25). This is the result of vacuum phenomenon, the same process found in the vertebral disc at a motion segment.

There is an increased chance of fracture at more than one level in the fused spine and the whole of the spine should be imaged, just as one would do with a long bone. MRI provides a reliable means of imaging the whole spine but this is not always possible in the severely kyphotic spine of a patient with AS who may not fit into the bore of an enclosed magnet.

NEUROLOGICAL INJURY

Spinal Cord

MRI provides an important prognostic indicator for neurological recovery following spinal cord injury. The

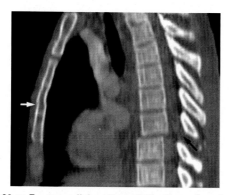

FIGURE 6-24 ■ **Fracture dislocation of the thoracic spine.** There is a step in the alignment and disruption across the spine with complete disruption of the posterior ligaments (note the 'epidural dirty fat' sign); there is an associated fracture of the sternum (arrow).

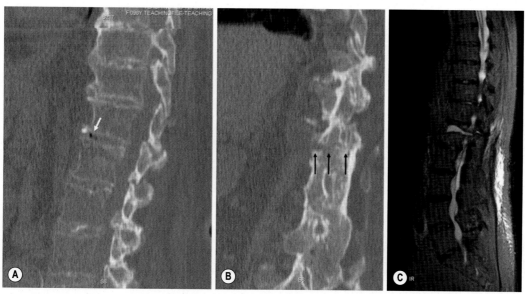

FIGURE 6-25 ■ **Fracture through the ankylosed spine in a patient with ankylosing spondylitis.** (A) The presence of vacuum phenomenon is evidence of spinal movement (arrow). (B) Sagittal CT through the facet joints. There is a faint fracture line (arrows) through the fused facet joints. (C) Sagittal STIR MRI demonstrates a fracture through the full width of the spine. The fracture through the vertebral body is difficult to define on CT, as the bone is very osteoporotic.

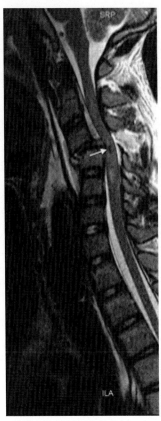

FIGURE 6-26 ■ Sagittal T2-weighted MRI. Low signal within the cord (arrow) is evidence of a cord haematoma. High signal inferior to this is cord oedema.

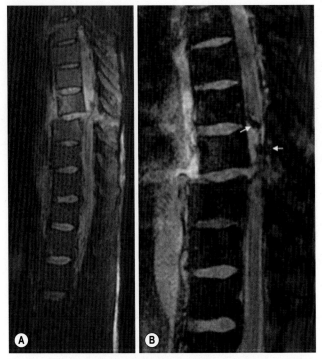

FIGURE 6-27 ■ Fracture dislocation with cord transection. (A) Sagittal STIR MRI and (B) gradient echo. The presence of blood is more clearly seen on the gradient echo sequence (arrows), which lies within the gap at the site of the cord transection.

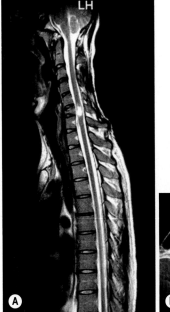
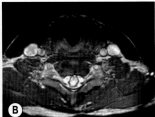

FIGURE 6-28 ■ Delayed post-traumatic spinal cord syrinx. T2-weighted MRI sagittal (A) and axial (B). A syrinx has developed at the site of previous spinal cord injury.

position of a burst fracture either above or below the level of the conus is important prognostically as trauma to the cauda equina has a much better neurological outcome than spinal cord injury. Mild cord oedema has a good prognosis for neurological improvement, whereas cord haemorrhage is a poor prognostic indicator and cord transection clearly has the worst prognosis. Haematomas within the cord less than 4 mm in diameter have a better neurological outcome than larger haemorrhages.[11]

In the acute setting haemorrhage within the cord will appear hypointense on T2-weighted turbo spin echo imaging due to the presence of deoxyhaemoglobin (Fig. 6-26). At a variable time after this, which may be up to 10 days, this becomes hyperintense due to the presence of methaemoglobin. The zone of hyperintensity begins at the periphery of the collection. None of these appearances will usually be confused with the uniform appearances of cord oedema, but gradient echo sequences can be used since these are more sensitive to the presence of haemorrhage (Fig. 6-27).

Delayed worsening of neurology after a spinal cord injury may be due to the development of a spinal cord syrinx (Fig. 6-28). Progressive enlargement of a syrinx can compromise the residual neurological function and surgical drainage of the syrinx may be required.

Brachial Plexus Injury

Nerve roots in the cervical spine can be avulsed from the cord, resulting in a brachial plexus injury. Whilst these commonly occur with an associated spinal injury in the

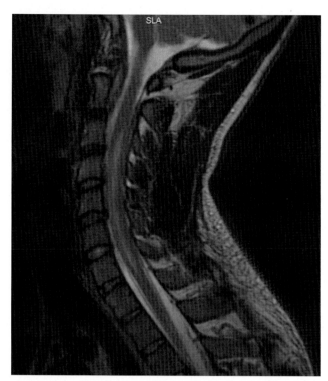

FIGURE 6-29 ■ **Sagittal T2-weighted MRI.** There is diffuse cord oedema due to nerve root avulsions at multiple levels.

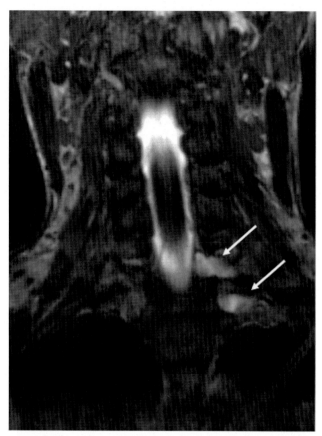

FIGURE 6-30 ■ **Coronal T2-weighted MRI 'myelogram' sequence.** Brachial plexus avulsion at C8 and T1 on the left with traumatic meningoceles (arrows).

polytrauma patient, the mechanism is one of a closed traction force applied to the shoulder and transmitted to the cord via the brachial plexus. Brachial plexus avulsion may be accompanied by diffuse spinal cord oedema, which should not be mistaken for the direct cord injury associated with a cervical spinal fracture (Fig. 6-29).

The lowest four cervical spinal nerves, C5–C8 and the first thoracic nerve T1 form the brachial plexus. Seventy-five per cent of cases of clinical brachial plexus injury involve avulsion of the roots from the cord[12] with 25 per cent confined to the distal brachial plexus.

MRI has largely replaced CT myelography in the diagnosis of nerve root avulsions with heavily T2-weighted 3D 'myelography' sequences, allowing the optimum slice orientation to demonstrate the intradural nerve roots. A complete nerve root avulsion is usually accompanied by a dural tear, resulting in a traumatic meningocele (Fig. 6-30). The demonstration of intact nerve roots in a patient with clinical brachial plexus injury suggests that the injury has occurred more distally within the brachial plexus, usually in the infraclavicular region.

REFERENCES

1. Henderson RL, Reid DC, Saboe LA. Multiple noncontiguous spine fractures. Spine 1991;16:128–31.
2. Ma R, Chow R, Shen FH. Kummell's disease: delayed post-traumatic osteonecrosis of the vertebral body. Eur Spine J 2010; 19:1065–70.
3. American College of Surgeons Committee on Trauma. Initial Assessment and Management. In: Advanced Trauma Life Support for Doctors. 8th ed. 2008. pp. 10.
4. Harris JH, Burke JT, Ray RD, et al. Low (type III) odontoid fracture: a new radiographic sign. Radiology 1984;153:353–6.
5. Denis F. The three column spine and its significance in the classification of acute thoracolumbar spinal injuries. Spine 1983;8: 817–31.
6. Oner FC, van Gils AP, Dhert WJ, Verbout AJ. MRI findings of thoracolumbar spine fractures: a categorisation based on MRI examinations of 100 fractures. Skeletal Radiol 1999;28: 433–43.
7. Magerl F, Aebi M, Gertzbein SD, et al. A comprehensive classification of thoracic and lumbar injuries. Eur Spine J 1994;3:184–201.
8. Chance GQ. Note on a type of flexion fracture of the spine. Br J Radiol 1948;21:452–3.
9. Wilcox RK, Boerger TO, Allen DJ, et al. A dynamic study of thoracolumbar burst fractures. J Bone Joint Surg Am 2003;85: 2184–9.
10. Boerger TO, Limb D, Dickson RA. Does 'canal clearance' affect neurological outcome after thoracolumbar burst fractures? J Bone Joint Surg Br 2000;82:629–35.
11. Boldin C, Raith J, Fankhauser F, et al. Predicting neurologic recovery in cervical spinal cord injury with postoperative MR imaging. Spine 2006;31:554–9.
12. Chuang DC. Management of traumatic brachial plexus injuries in adults. Hand Clin 1999;15:737–55.

Page numbers followed by '*f*' indicate figures, '*t*' indicate tables, and '*b*' indicate boxes.

susceptibility artefacts, 16
three-dimensional imaging, 15
truncation artefacts, 16
myelography, 8–10, 9f
contraindications, 9
pre-imaging screening, 9
radiography, 6–8
disadvantage, 6
full AP view, 8, 8f
functional lateral views, 7f, 8
trauma, 6
Spinocerebellar ataxia, 89
Spinous processes
degenerative changes, 34, 34f
spinal anatomy, 2f–3f, 3
Spondylodiscitis, 95–96
Spondylolisthesis, 34–35, 34f
Spondylosis deformans, 19, 20f
Stenosis
failed back surgery syndrome, 98–99, 99f
Sterile arachnoiditis, failed back surgery
syndrome, 98, 98f
STIR see Short-tau inversion recovery (STIR)
Subacute combined degeneration of the
spinal cord (SCD), 89, 89f
Subarticular intervertebral disc herniation,
23, 27f
Superior articular process, facet joints, 3
Supraspinous ligament, 5
Susceptibility artefacts, spine MRI, 16
Synovial cysts, postoperative, 99f
Synthetic bone grafts, spinal cord
stabilisation, 91–92, 92f
Syringomyelia, 86f, 87–88
Systemic lupus erythematosus (SLE), 72–73
MRI, 72–73, 75f

T

Taenia solium infection see Cysticercosis;
Neurocysticercosis
Tarlov cysts (perineural arachnoid cysts), 87
Thoracic spine
intervertebral disc annular tears, 22
myelography, 10

radiography, 6–7
trauma frequency, 102
Thoracolumbar junction
trauma frequency, 102
Thoracolumbar spine, 106
CT, 106
radiographs, 106
Thoracolumbar spine trauma, 110–115
burst fractures, 112–114
AP radiograph, 112, 114f
axial CT, 114
kyphosis, 114
pincer burst fracture, 114
classification systems, 110–114
AO classification system, 110
MRI, 110
flexion compression/distraction injuries,
111–112, 111f–112f
Chance fractures, 111–112, 113f
kyphosis, 112, 113f
soft-tissue Chance fractures, 111–112
fracture dislocation, 114–115, 115f
TLIF (transforaminal lumbar interbody
fusion), 92
Transforaminal lumbar interbody fusion
(TLIF), 92
Transverse ligament, craniocervical junction,
5
Transverse processes, spinal anatomy, 2f–3f,
3
Transverse tears, intervertebral discs, 21
Truncation artefacts, spine MRI, 16
Tuberculosis
spinal cord infection, 80–81, 82f
Tumefactive multiple sclerosis, 73f

V

Varicella-zoster virus (VZV) infection
spinal cord, 81
Vascular endothelial growth factor (VEGF),
48
Vasculature
non-tumoural spinal cord lesions,
76–80

VEGF (vascular endothelial growth factor),
48
Vertebrae
body, 1, 2f
endplate changes see Vertebral endplate
changes
osteomyelitis see Vertebral osteomyelitis
Vertebral endplate changes, 23–25
bone marrow modic changes, 25
subchondral bone, 23–24, 25t
type 1 changes, 24, 29f
type 2 changes, 24, 29f
type 3 changes, 24
Vertebral osteomyelitis
spinal surgery complications, 95–96, 95f
Vertebral tumours
benign
aneurysmal bone cysts, 41f, 60–61
eosinophilic granuloma, 61–62, 61f
haemangioma, 57–58, 58f–59f
osteoblastoma, 58, 59f, 60
osteoid osteoma, 58, 59f
locally aggressive, 63–65
chordoma, 63–64, 63f–64f
giant cell tumours, 41f, 64–65, 64f
primary malignant, 65–68
chondrosarcoma, 41f, 66
Ewing's sarcoma, 66–67
multiple myeloma, 65–66, 65f–66f
osteosarcoma, 67–68, 68f
plasmacytoma, 65–66
Vertebrectomy, 91
Vertebroplasty
image-guided percutaneous bone
augmentation, 99–100, 100f
Viral myelitis, 81, 83f
Von Hippel–Lindau syndrome
spinal haemangioma, 46–48, 48f
VZV see Varicella-zoster virus (VZV)
infection

W

World Health Organization (WHO)
spinal tumour classification, 43–44

Printed in the United States
By Bookmasters